Not Just The Cleaning Lady:

A Hygienist's Guide to Survival

Not Just The Cleaning Lady:

A Hygienist's Guide to Survival

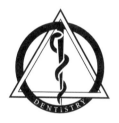

Cat A. Schmidt, RDH

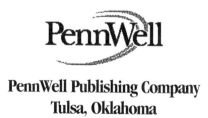

PennWell Publishing Company
Tulsa, Oklahoma

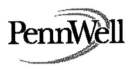

PennWell Publishing
Tulsa, Oklahoma

Copyright (c) 1997 by
PennWell Publishing Company
1421 South Sheridan/P.O. Box 1260
Tulsa, Oklahoma 74101

Schmidt, Catherine A.
    Not just the cleaning lady : a hygienist's guide to survival /
Catherine A. Schmidt.
       p. cm.
    Includes bibliographical references and index.
    ISBN 0-8714-672-5
    1. Dental hygiene--Vocational guidance.   I. Title.
    [DNLM: 1. Dental Hygienists.   2. Dental Care--organization &
    administration.   3. Dental Assistants.   WU 90 S349n 1997]
RK60.5.S335   1997
617.6'01'023--dc21
DNLM/DLC
for Library of Congress   97-47790
                                                  CIP

Printed in the United States of America

1 2 3 4 5 01 00 99 98 97

Dedicated to Papa and Dianne,
Cyd and David, and Mother,
who teach me daily
that through God, all things are possible.

Table of Contents

Acknowledgments vii

Preface ix

Introduction xii

Chapter 1   I Do Windows:
            Accepting Computerization 1

Chapter 2   Covering Your Assets: Insurance
            and Legal Issues 25

Chapter 3   Infection Protection: OSHA Comes
            Calling 45

Chapter 4   The Next Generation: Hygiene Assistants
            and Assistance 67

Chapter 5   Patients of the Millennium: Defining
            and Treating Geriatric Patients....................................83

Chapter 6   The Invisible Uniform: A Refresher
            Course in Professionalism 95

Chapter 7   Not Just the Cleaning Lady: Synthesizing
            Hygiene with Dentistry 121

Chapter 8   Back in the Saddle: Re-entering the Work
            Force or Switching Offices 139

Postscript   Coffee Breaks: Taking Time for You...............................151

References 159
Index 161

Acknowledgments

Thank you to the following who contributed generously to this book:

Access, magazine of the ADHA

The American Dental Hygienists' Association
444 N. Michigan Ave., Ste. 3400
Chicago, IL 60611
1-800-243-2342

Robert Ankrom, RDH, BS, Consultant, McKenzie Management

AOL/RDH e-mailers

Phyllis Beemsterboer, RDH, Ed.D., ADHA Commissioner
to the ADA Commission on Dental Accreditation; Acting Assistant
Dean, Administration Affairs, UCLA School of Dentistry.

Kirk Bjornsgaard, Editor, PennWell Publishing

Kathy Eklund, RDH, MHP, Clinical Associate Professor
Forsyth School for Dental Hygienists; Infection Control Consultant for the
Boston Public Health Commission

Team Gentle Dental, for teaching me how to work together to provide
excellent dentistry, and to have fun in the process:
Hygiene: **Patti, Eileen, Barb, Allison H., Deb A., and Robin.**
Dentists: **Schmidty, Jim, Masih, and Jeff.**
Lab: **Dionne, Mary, John, Shawn, and Deb T.**
Business: **Doris, Marcia, Jean, Debbie C., Stef B., Cathie, Amy, Allison B.,
and LeAnn.**
Assisting: **Debbie R., Kim, Sarah, Jeannie, Carla, Rhonda, Heide, Trudi,
Diana, and Tammy.**
Sterilization: **Pam and Ann.**

Cindy Girard, RDH

Mark Hartley, Editor, PennWell Publishing

JADA (Journal of the American Dental Association)
Journal of Practical Hygiene

Acknowledgments

Ann Kinney, Illusions Photography

Sandra Leggett, RDH, MA, Des Moines Area Community College

Maria McKenzie, RDH, BA, MS, an ADHA president, adjunct faculty University of California, San Francisco, and lecturer on women's health

John McPherson, "Close to Home"

New Hampshire Technical Institute Dental Hygiene Department

Jill Nield-Gehring, RDH, MA

Lisa Paschang, RDH, MPA

PennWell Publishing
RDH: The National Magazine for Dental Hygiene Professionals

Sarah Turner, RDH, MEd, Hawkeye Community College; Former ADHA President.

Dr. Richard Simms, DDS, MS

Steve Smith, DDS, MS; **Rick Green**, DDS; and **Patrick McKenna**, DMD

Virginia Woodward, RDH, Executive Director for the Kentucky Commission on Women; Former ADHA President

Cyd, for our sister weekends and entrepreneurial dreams.

David, for San Fran tours and sharing Cyd.

Mom, for "why not?" breaks and dinners.

Papa, for MNF, lunches, and my lifelong association with dentistry.

Dianne, for really cool cards and taking care of Schmidt-Dog.

Toodles, for your twisted sense of humor.

Patti and Bill, for renting homes and, "Keep your stick on the ice!"

Ken for pizza and cheap seats movies.

Joni, **Dana** and **Jean** for not making me walk the plank.

The Williams Gang, for the laugh track.

The Griggs Clan, for guiding me through the storm.

And, finally, an apple for each of my school teachers.

Preface

Three thousand years ago, an Egyptian woman lived along the lush, fruitful river Nile. Pyramids dotted the outlying desert landscape, built by rulers whom she knew as gods: the Pharaohs. Her name was Djedmaatesankh—Djed for short—and she was the Harriet Nelson of her time, a middle-class housewife.

One hot, mosquito-ridden night, Djed awoke with a toothache. The throbbing in her head was immense. She lay awake until dawn, when her husband finally insisted she see the doctor. Physicians who specialized in teeth were scarce, but luckily there was one in her city.

Dentistry, as a branch of medicine, has been around since 2500 B.C. That's the year the first dentist of record is mentioned. His name was Hesi-Re and his ruler was King Zoser, who requisitioned construction of the Step Pyramid, most likely the first pyramid built in Egypt. Hesi-Re predated Djed by 1500 years, so dentistry was already an ancient science by the time Djed awoke with her toothache.

Djed made her way grudgingly to the tooth doctor. Peering inside her mouth, he saw a fistula above the aching tooth. He smiled reassuringly and proceeded to drill a hole into the side of the jawbone, thus providing a drainage canal for the fluid. This brought instant relief for Djed, as the pain from the pressure subsided.

The doctor patted her hand, and advised her to mix one part cumin, one part incense and one part onion into a paste and apply it to the tooth. This, he assured her, would cure the bad tooth. He sent her on her way, back to her home and husband and duties. A week later, Djed died. The cause of death, perhaps undetermined at the time, was from a dental abscess.

A few years ago, Djed's tomb was found on a routine excavation in Egypt. Her sarcophagus, or crypt, contained all the information about her life. Where she lived, the name and position of her husband and notable events that affected her brief stay on Earth. This find was most unusual in the fact that Djed was an ordinary citizen. She was not a queen or a high priestess. She was a normal, average person, just like you and me. She had hopes and dreams and fears. She lived simply and plainly in an ancient world that now evokes images of mysticism and treasure.

It's interesting to think of Djed and wonder what someone would think of us 3,000 years from now. Let's say in the fifth millennium they opened up a twenty-first century crypt. Would they think it odd if the person had died of cancer, or in a car accident, or from a virus? ("Mommy, why did she die from a virus?" "Because, honey, they didn't have the vaccine back then.")

What was Djed's legacy? What will be ours? Our time on this planet is but a millisecond in history. Our lifelong joys, dreams, triumphs, and disappointments begin with our birth and usually end with our passing. A few have left an indelible mark on history, and these great men and women live in our history books, science books and in literature. But in greater numbers, sometimes people just as great enter and leave this world with nothing more than a few announcements in a local newspaper.

It is said that 100 years from today it does not matter what kind of car we drove, or the size of the diamond sitting on our finger, but what will matter is the impact we've had on the life of a child. Our lasting footprint upon the earth is the difference each of us makes in the lives of others. Who we touch, what we do, how we live determines our legacy. A legacy is both a treasure and a burden to be revered.

We may have first learned about legacy as children. I remember first thinking about legacy in elementary school when we scrawled our names in the chipping paint of the lavatory stalls. Temporary, sure, but still our "marks" were these scratches left for the future. This was part of us that could survive and tell others that we were once here.

My lasting impression of legacy came in the form of a time capsule. Back in the early 1970s, a popular activity was to create time capsules. It seems everyone thought they were living in special times and wanted to capture it for future generations (as if posterity would be interested in wide polyester ties and pet rocks 100 years hence).

Our class convened to choose contemporary items for our special time capsule. We were so proud of our decisions of what should be passed along to future generations, none of which I distinctly remember now, of course. The items included a newspaper, a magazine and some toys. The biggest item was a tape recording of our voices with comments on the events of the times. An audiotape, not video. There were no video cameras back then.

Video was a new entity. No videos, no camcorders, no video stores. If you missed the movie in the theater, you missed it altogether. My parents owned one of the first Betamax's in our city. Sitting atop our console television set, the Betamax was a huge, ugly, foreign contraption. It forced the moving of framed family pictures to other tabletops. Using large, bulky Betamax tapes, we recorded early '70's television shows, the names of which—thankfully—I have long since banished from my memory.

Recording Christmas holidays or Halloween tricks and treats to watch on the Beta was never a thought. Camcorders were a decade away from the grasping hands of the mass market. Special events were filmed using Dad's 8-mm camera. In making our time capsule, I suppose our class could have used that classic 8-mm film to capture our polyester-clad images for the "future" we were assured would provide us with technological convenience and ample time for leisure activities. But tape recorders were readily available from the audio/video department, so we used audiotapes. Our giggly, whiny screams permanently imprinted on a strip of plastic for future generations to ponder, "What imbecile gave these kids a microphone?"

Once in a great while, when the smell of summer hits me just right as I pass a group of children inline skating on the blacktop of an elementary schoolyard, I wonder whatever happened to that time capsule. As I recall, we buried it on school grounds near a struggling sapling. They've probably placed a new gym over it by now, sealing it for the new century. Just as well. If they brought it up in my lifetime, I'd have to own up to it. And I want my legacy to be a little more than a Partridge Family album and a United States bicentennial silver dollar.

Our daily lives are a lot like that time capsule. Every time we touch another person we place another item in our time capsule, creating a legacy of our choosing. We, as dental hygienists, are born nurturers. Our livelihoods are mere extensions of our inner selves, desiring to heal and teach. Our professional legacy is the patience, guidance, and care we provide our patients, co-workers and employers.

Introduction

"When a just cause reaches its flood tide...
whatever stands in the way must fall before its overwhelming power."

—Carrie Chapman Catt
from a speech at Stockholm,
Is Woman Suffrage Progressing?

Out of hygiene school we pop, ready to tackle the work of periodontal disease. Armed with a scaler and books of knowledge, we feel certain to win each and every battle for complete oral health. We are saviors, tackling every unflossed, plaque-filled, grungy mouth with vigor.

Then—boom!—it hits. Smack in the face like a bonk between the eyes: reality.

Your boss wants you to help the receptionist file charts. Your patients give the "I-could-not-care-less" look after you skillfully demonstrate the fine art of Modified Bass. The office gets a new computer. You hear about the hygienist who had her license yanked because her dentist submitted costly perio codes to insurance for child prophys. The Occupational Safety and Health Administration (OSHA) visits and wants to interview you.

In other words, you've discovered there's more to hygiene than calculus removal and a nice paycheck. There are patients who threaten to sue, dentists who wish to have auxiliaries perform hygiene duties, and computers that crash. Maybe a co-worker won't stop gossiping about a colleague, or the pressures of work are creeping into home life.

It's a cold, cruel world out there. How can you keep your focus on performing well when the roadblocks of dental business slow you down? What information regarding OSHA, computers, insurance, hygiene assistants and professionalism is imperative for you to know? How can you promote yourself to get the hygiene job of your dreams? What is managed care and how will it affect your practice? What are the trends in dental hygiene after the millennium?

It's all summarized here in these few pages. Each chapter is designed to give you insight into specific areas that affect your job, your career, yourself. This book will allow you to successfully reap the benefits of a long, rewarding hygiene career and keep your cool during high-pressure situations.

After all, we're more than just cleaning ladies.

Chapter One

I Do Windows: Accepting Computerization

"No idea is so antiquated that it was not once modern. No idea is so modern that it will not someday be antiquated."

> –Ellen Glasgow
> from *Address to the Modern Language Society* (1936)

Teaching Old Dogs New Tricks

On a cold, winter evening in 1938, in a dimly-lit tavern in the Midwest, John Vincent Atanasoff, a professor at Iowa State University, invented the computer. Later called the ABC, for Atanasoff-Berry Computer, after the inventor and his assistant, it was perhaps the most stunning invention of the twentieth century.[1] Today we take computers for granted, and wonder how we could survive without them, yet they are mostly unnoticed, helpful additions to our lives. Computers pop up everywhere. They make things happen faster, better, and more accurately.

It's easy to see the ways we use computers every day. We use computers when we make phone calls, complete credit card transactions, purchase items at a store, drive a new car, fly in an airplane, or watch cable television. And that's just the tip of the iceberg. Computers are literally everywhere in our lives, becoming practically mandatory to daily function.

So why are they so intimidating? Because anything new is intimidating.

When automatic teller machine keypads were first installed at grocery stores and gas stations, we didn't know how to use them. But, after years of using that magic card swipe and feeling comfortable paying for our food and petrol without writing a check, we adapted to the point of no return. Through use grows acceptance.

The same is true for computers in dental offices. Our co-workers and patients can be daunted by computers and so can we, especially since this is relatively virgin ground for computers. We're at the threshold of computer use in dental offices. This is catching some of us off-guard.

"I almost quit," says Pearl, a hygienist in New Hampshire. "When my dentist said we were getting computers, I thought, this is it. I'm out of here."

So, Pearl gave her notice and planned a departure date. During that time, however, computer training began in the office, and terminals popped up in the operatories and at the front desk. Files and charts disappeared as they were scanned into the new system. Pearl was forced to use the computer to perform her job in the last weeks.

"I had a horrible attitude. I didn't care to learn it because I was leaving. But then, well, I just had to use it. Flo, our receptionist, couldn't help me when we were busy, so I had to learn to do things on my own. Pretty soon it became easier."

Pearl started with a few simple tasks at first—entering charges, then ledger notes. Soon, she picked up charting and prescriptions. "We didn't have prescription pads anymore. It was all on computer. So, if my patient needed Peridex, I had to ask an assistant to do it for me. If she was tied up, I fell behind. Finally, I asked her to show me how. It was difficult at first, but I did it, all on my own," she glows.

Pearl's experiences are not uncommon. Generally, when people are in a situation that they must do or die, they will do. Pearl didn't want to learn to use the computer, but given no alternative to seeing or dismissing patients, she learned to use it. In fact, by the time she had scheduled to leave, her computer skills were up to par with others in the office. Her dentist asked her stay on, and, after some soul searching, she decided to take him up on the offer. She and the new hire now work together as part of a computerized dental office.

Not all situations turn out as well as Pearl's did. It takes time, patience (more on that later), determination, and a real desire to learn to use computers in a dental setting. When our office first became fully computerized, way back in 1990, two of 24 employees did not stay through training. It's not for everyone. But it is for anyone who desires to make the effort.

Sophia works for a periodontist in Chicago. Her knowledge of computers was zero the day her dentist brought in Computerized Dental Radiography (CDR). Sophia takes bitewings and full mouth series (FMS) many times throughout the day. She was really frightened of computerized x-rays, as most of us would be. Attaching a computer to something as sensitive and imperative to dentistry as radiographs intensifies the effect. Without x-rays the dental profession flies blind. When a computer takes over the film and developing technique, nerves are bound to rattle a bit.

"It took me 55 minutes to do one full mouth series the first time I used it," she says in a sweet, German accent. "I thought the patient was going to walk out on me." Sophia never considered leaving the office. She was bound and determined to make the CDR work, or convince her employer to get rid of it. She watched the accompanying video three times and practiced on each patient who needed an FMS. Either she'd understand it, or the computer was going to go.

"My time got shorter and shorter. In weeks, I could do full mouth exposures in 12 minutes," she explains. "I like it, now." Sophia learned practice makes perfect. Her best asset was desire to learn. Through that she was able to reach her goal and learn the computer. Determination is the first step in conquering computer phobia.

Keystrokes for All Folks

It's not a surprise to anyone that, if you've grown up with computers in your home, school, or your daily life, that computers will not pose a threat. If you've always had computers, you accept them. You know that each one functions differently, so you just need to learn the specifics on each program on each computer. A new computer in your dental office won't throw you for a loop, because you understand the basics.

But what if computers are new to you? Let's say you didn't grow up with computers, or you don't use them frequently at home, in school or even at the gas station. Does merely mentioning the word "computer" throw you into a tizzy? Your hands sweat, your pulse races and you long for a paper chart and a blue and red pencil. It's okay, there's hope for you.

Gloria's employer told her they were going to computerize the office. Not just add a computer, but fully computerize the office. That included everything—charts, files, records, x-rays, the whole nine yards. Gloria panicked, because she'd never used a computer before, and quite frankly, didn't think she could.

But Gloria's son, a computer genius at age 9 (all 9-year-olds are computer geniuses), encouraged her. "Mom, you can do it. Everyone uses computers. It's really easy." Gloria wasn't so sure, but she figured if a 9-year-old can learn it, then at least she could do a half-Aztec job. So, why not give it a try?

Gloria's first lesson consisted of learning how to turn on and off the system. The more complicated the system, the more important this function is. There are certain ways to turn on and off a computer. It's not as simple as flicking a switch. It's like getting the computer ready for bed: wash its face, brush its teeth, say its prayers, and tuck it in. The procedure is methodical and repetitious. The rule is to just follow this course, step by step, and learn it by rote.

Learning to turn the computer on and off is like learning to wear a seat belt. Remember when most states passed seat belt laws (those of us who are old enough!)? Some of us needed to learn to wear one. Every time we got in the car, we consciously reminded ourselves to put on our seat belts. By putting it on each time, we made it part of our "car routine." Pretty soon, it became habit. Clicking on the right icons and turning off the right switches to shut down the computer after a while becomes habit. It's just something you do when you're finished for the day.

As with learning anything new, it takes a while to get past the point where it's a concentrated effort. While you're learning, you'll burn a lot

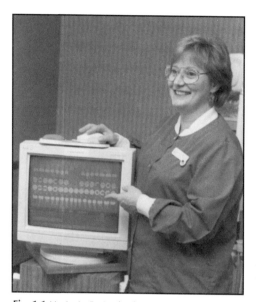

Fig. 1.1 Hygienist Patti Ireland uses the mouse with Chartit, a computer charting program.

of mental calories consciously thinking about each and every step. Over time, and with practice, those same actions will become second nature. Your fingers will move to the place that you need them without concerted brain drain.

The same was true for Gloria. One day, she shut down the computer and didn't think about each step. She just did it. It had become second nature. Practice makes perfect...or at least, makes it easier. And practice is the key to learning computers. It takes time, energy and effort to learn to use a computer. It's not easy—nothing worthwhile ever is—but the benefits are enormous. The time and energy saved in the long run is worth the initiation process.

Gloria was lucky because she was in a practice that excelled in computer training. They shut down for a few days to really give the employees time to adjust and learn. Gloria took it step by step. She knew she wasn't going to learn it overnight, but she also knew she had to keep trying. She started with the basic functions. She spent an hour playing with the mouse, learning to click, double click, drag, and highlight. Pretty soon, she was feeling comfortable. Most computers contain tutorials that guide the user through separate computer functions, such as a mouse tutorial. Utilizing these tutorials is a helpful introduction to the computer.

"I'd never touched a mouse before. It was strange. It took me awhile to realize that if it went off the screen, and I was at the edge of my pad, that all I had to do was lift the mouse and replace. I felt really good when I figured that out." (Fig. 1.1.)

Not everyone is able to jump in and learn all the keystrokes they need in one day. Learning to integrate computers into your dental routine takes patience. At first, everything will take longer, as the office adjusts to new routines. Every team member will be thinking consciously about what she is doing, which can be exhausting. The period of adjustment can take days or weeks, but the results will be favorably noticeable, as tasks become easier and quicker over time. The office mindset must be that in the long run everyone will benefit.

"Once I got the hang of the computer, I was able to cut down my charting time," says Gloria. She learned that computers can save time filing and retrieving data. Though initially computers zap us of time and energy, the pay-off does come. And it comes big, with more efficient use of time, easier retrieval of data, and more patient information available with the touch of a key on the keyboard.

Her old way of entering info on the chart was to write: "Adult Prophy, Bitewing X-rays, Fluoride Treatment, POH Instruction, Periodic Oral Exam. Patient presented with slight to moderate calculus, good POH, needs to floss more. Recommend six-month recall to maintain oral health."

Her new way to enter info on the computer was: "C-enter-ABF." "N-enter- P6." (Fig 1.2.) These are called explosion codes. Explosion codes are computer shorthand. They are a quick way to enter information without having to type every word. For specifics, Gloria could jump to another screen and type, "Slight to moderate calculus, good POH, needs to floss more, going to Europe in August." She's got the repetitive text in shorthand. She can type the specifics in a narrative style.

Explosion codes save time. When one types in "C" (for "complete") then strokes the Enter key and types "CF" (for child prophy with periodic oral exam and fluoride), the computer records that the hygienist has just completed a child prophy with exam and fluoride treatment.

This action places the charges on the child's record, which is linked to all other family members. The computer automatically bills the parent, not the child. In our office we expect payment upon delivery of service, so billing is not an expected function, but since there are no absolutes in life, billing does happen. The procedures are also dated so that for the next visit, the hygienist or dentist can easily see what was completed at the last appointment.

As soon as the charges are keyed in, the computer calculates the

Computer Explosion Codes
(These are the ones chosen in my office; they will differ system to system,
office to office.)

Type of explosion code:
C = Completed Treatment on Patient (charged out).
N = Notes (we have a stock of preselected notes to use).
T = Treatment Recommended for patient (not charged out).

Here's a sampling of explosion codes we use in our office. These are hygiene relevant:
A = Adult Prophy, Periodic Oral Exam.
AB = Adult Prophy, Bitewing X rays, Periodic Oral Exam.
ABF = Adult Prophy, Bitewing X rays, Fluoride Treatment, Periodic Oral Exam.
ABFP = Adult Prophy, Bitewing X rays, Fluoride, Panoramic X ray, Periodic Oral Exam.
Y = Youth Prophy, Periodic Oral Exam.
YB = Youth Prophy, Bitewing X rays, Periodic Oral Exam.
YBF = Youth Prophy, Bitewing X rays, Fluoride Treatment, Periodic Oral Exam.
YBFP = Youth Prophy, Bitewing X rays, Fluoride, Panoramic X ray, Periodic Oral Exam.
C = Child Prophy, Periodic Oral Exam.
CB = Child Prophy, Bitewing X rays, Periodic Oral Exam.
CBF = Child Prophy, Bitewing X rays, Fluoride Treatment, Periodic Oral Exam.
CBFP = Child Prophy, Bitewing X rays, Fluoride, Panoramic X ray, Periodic Oral Exam.
BW2C = Bitewing X rays Computer Digitized Radiography.
BW2 = Bitewing Xrays Celluloid Film.
DENT = Dentin Bloc Desensitizer applied.
EX = Initial Exam, Operatory.
EXH = Inital Exam, Hygiene.
EXHT = Initial Exam, Title XIX.
EXPH = Periodic Oral Exam, Regular and Title XIX.
FTA = Fluoride Treatment Adult.
FTC = Fluoride Treatment Child.
PA1C = Periapical X ray Computer Digitized Radiography.
PAN = Panoramic X ray.
PLAT = Platinum Whitening System.
PM1 = Premed taken one hour before appointment.
PM2 = Will take premed six hours after initial dose.
PREV = Prevident Fluoride Gel, one tube.
PROBC = Complete Periodontal Probe Performed.
PROPH = Adult Prophy age 18 and up.
PROPY = Youth Prophy age 15 and up.
PROCH = Child Prophy through age 14.
PROPJ = Title XIX Adult Prophy Fluoride age 13 and up.
PROCJ = Title XIX Child Prophy Fluoride through age 12.
PROP1 = First Prophy.
PROP2 = Second Prophy.
RPQ = Root Plane Quadrant.
RPQ- = Root Plane Less Than Quadrant.
RP2+ = Root Plane A Few Teeth.
For PSR scores: enter "C," then enter the score (i.e., "1"), then enter the
sextant (i.e., "6").

Fig 1.2 Typical explosion codes

insurance and patient portions of the invoice. The front desk knows immediately what the patient owes, if anything. This speeds check-out and ultimately helps with collections. With a few keystrokes the receptionist can hand a receipt to the parent, and say, "Your insurance covers 90 percent of Brianna's cleaning today. Your portion is seven dollars."

For notes, type "N" (for "notes") hit Enter, then type "PA" (for "parental approval"). The PA note says, "Obtained parental permission for procedures performed today." Then, type "N" again, and hit Enter followed by "PP" (for "pedo prophy"). The PP note says: "Polish and floss. Reviewed home care, brushing and/or flossing with patient and/or parent. Recommended 6 (six)-month recall to maintain dental health. Examining dentist reports oral cancer screening exam negative." On another screen, I might add my own words: "Brianna was great helper! Mom is helping with brushing a.m. and p.m. Dr. Knight wants to keep close watch for ortho referral."

Those few keystrokes create a permanent, unalterable, dated record. This is great news for those of us who think in terms of legal issues. There can be no dispute over what we said happened in our office today. A year down the line we might not remember the exact appointment, but with dated, complete notes, we are reminded. (Fig. 1.3.)

Explosion codes offer a quick alternative to longhand. Why is this important? So we can spend more time at the chair, interacting with our patients.

> **Computers free us of time-consuming tasks, so we can spend more time with our patients.**

The EDO

There are three stages of dental office computerization. The first stage is what's called the financial stage. All the office finances are placed on computer. This rarely has a direct effect on patient care delivery. It means that billing, accounts receivable/payable, taxes, payroll, and such are done on computer. These systems can link to insurance companies, credit bureaus, and other out-of-office resources.

The second stage is partial computerization. This is where most office systems are handled by computers. All finances are manipulated and stored by computer, along with patient files that contain such information as medical history, clinic notes, family data, and charges. Usually there are links to the outside world for insurance claims and credit card processing.

The third stage is nearly complete computerization. Named the Electronic Dental Office (EDO) by Duane A. Schmidt, DDS, in his book, *Schmidt's Anatomy of a Successful Dental Practice*, published by PennWell Publishing in 1996, this is an office where most systems are handled by computer. There are no paper records of

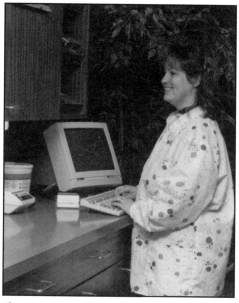

Fig. 1-3
Assistant Deb Rassler enters ledger notes on a patient after the patient has been dismissed.

any kind kept. Everyone in the office uses computers for one purpose or another. It is a fully integrated system.

Let me show you how an EDO works by following Gary, a first-time patient in our office. Computer systems used in this office are Dentech, Chart-it, Schick's Computer Digitized Radiography, and other systems and programs for billing, taxes, and finances that I won't mention here because they're not relevant to hygiene.

"Gary #1"

Gary enters the navy blue and maroon waiting area through a glass door. He heads to the reception desk and gives his name to Darlene, the receptionist. This is Gary's first visit to an EDO.

Darlene welcomes him with a warm smile and asks him to take a seat by the patient registration computer. She enters "moni" on her computer, which pulls up the monitor program. With two keystrokes Darlene "sends" Gary's arrival time back to the hygiene room. The hygienist, Ellen, can check the computer monitor mounted on the wall, to see that Gary arrived at 9:55 a.m.

The monitor is a lot like arrival and departure monitors in airports. The monitor will show Gary's provider initials and the time of his scheduled appointment, followed by his name (last/first), and then his arrival time and the number of minutes either before or after his scheduled appointment time. When Gary shows on the monitor, his line will read: "EH 10:00 MEINIKE, GAR 9:55 5." The monitor has only so many spaces for a name, so sometimes the first name is incomplete. This is never a problem since an appointment schedule sheet (for provider EH: Ellen Hart) is available for cross reference. Since Gary is five minutes early, the minute marker will read five, then four, then three, two, one, until 10:00 a.m. Then it will begin a cycle again, this time showing the minutes after his appointment: one, two, three and so on.

Knowing that Gary is a "number one," or new patient, Ellen knows she has time to wrap up her current patient before Gary will be ready. Ellen's assistant places a red check over Gary's name on the appointment schedule sheet. That way, anyone who glances at Ellen's schedule will know Gary has arrived, even after her assistant has taken him off the monitor with a keystroke.

Removing Gary from the monitor allows room for the rest of the day's appointments. Each appointment appears on the monitor 30 minutes before the scheduled arrival time. So if another hygienist had an appointment at 10:30, her patient would come into view at 10:00 a.m., perhaps reading: "TW 10:30 GEISEL, THEO 30," for a Theodore Geisel at 10:30 a.m. with Tammi Woo.

If a patient does not show up on time, the word "LATE" appears behind the name followed by the minutes that patient is late. If Ted (Theodore) were to be late, his line would read: "TW 10:30 GEISEL, THEO LATE 3." Tammi then can take action. When the late minutes read 10, she will phone Ted at home to see if his wife says he's on his way, or if he's home and forgot his appointment and needs to reschedule. When the minutes read 15, and she hasn't been able to contact Ted, Tammi will intercom (on the privacy of a phone, not a speaker) and tell Darlene to "BA" Ted. A BA is a broken appointment.

Back at Ellen's current appointment, Gary is up at the front desk reading a health history questionnaire on a computer screen. The screen is touch sensitive, so Gary presses his finger on each situation that relates to his medical condition. Darlene guides him through every screen as Gary reads and makes the necessary selections. She hands him a plastic stick shaped like a pen and Gary scribes his signature directly

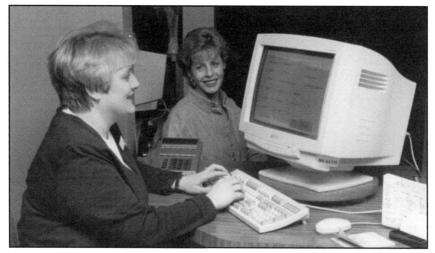

Fig. 1-4 Receptionist Stef Breslin initializes the health history touch screen for patient Robin Clark.

onto the screen. (Fig. 1.4.) His signature states that his medical history is accurate as entered, that he will allow us to release his dental treatment information for third-party reimbursement, and that he agrees to the terms of binding arbitration (more on this in Chapter 2).

Signatures on computers are considered legal and valid. Programs that store signatures have special protectors built so that alteration is not possible, which explains why these programs are in use everywhere, from store credit card transactions to shipping company deliveries. All fully-computerized companies require computerized signatures. It's not the wave of the future, it's here and now.

After Darlene obtains his signature, she asks Gary to have a seat in the waiting room. While he's watching television or reading, she enters his vital medical history, such as medications and health conditions, onto an electronic chart. She then prints out a Patient Care Form (PCF) for Ellen. In big, black letters at the top she writes: "Gary #1." (Fig. 1.5.) If his wife were due that day, she'd print one for her and write "Maggie" at the top. (Fig. 1.6.)

A PCF is a piece or two of paper that contains important information about the patient. It's like a temporary chart, used just for one appointment before it's shredded and recycled. Ellen uses a PCF as a quick reference guide for pertinent medical, insurance, and dental information. If she needs more detailed data on Gary she can check the computer.

The PCF shows Ellen nearly all the material she'll need on Gary for that appointment. Gary is allergic to ampicillin and codeine, so Darlene will have highlighted that info in pink. All pertinent medical information including prescribed medicines will appear smack dab in the middle of the first page. Easy to read, easy to see. If carbocaine is indicated it will be noted there, with Darlene's pink highlighter ensuring it's read. Premedication information would be in the same place, highlighted in pink and noted also on the appointment schedule sheet at the front desk, as well as on the copy in the hygiene room. Both Darlene and Ellen will ask if premed has been taken for the day's procedures. Double-checks like this assure no mistakes are made.

Since Gary is new to the office, his past appointment information will be blank. For each patient, the dates of last prophy, visit, bitewing, panoramic x-ray (pan), denture, and reline will appear under each column, as well as one for each member of the family. That way, both staff and Gary can see when his wife last visited the office, and when her bitewings and pan were taken.

We use that feature at every appointment to check for need of bitewings and pan. One glance and we know when the last ones were taken. Gary, as a number-one patient, will probably need bitewings, and maybe a pan.

Ellen takes him into the x-ray room. She places a Computer Digitized Radiography (CDR) sensor in his mouth and snaps the picture. Instantly, the image is projected onto a computer monitor on the wall. It shows a perfect bitewing. She takes the mate, and a pan, and walks him to her chair in the hygiene room.

When she's settled, her assistant, Cydney, comes over for charting. Cydney brings up Chart-it on the large monitor at the foot of the chair. Ellen calls out the restoration and periodontal pocket data to Cydney, and, presto, Ellen has all the information she needs at her fingertips.

Cydney pulls up the CDR program that displays Gary's bitewings. With the click of a mouse, Ellen can switch among the screen showing restorations, the screen showing probing depths, and the screens showing bitewings and pan. When the doctor comes over for the full exam, he can flip through these screens to get a good picture of Gary's oral health.

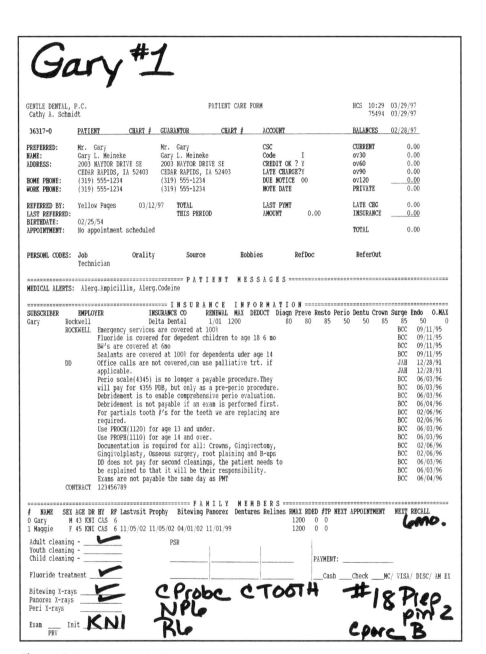

Figure 1.5 Patient Care Form for Gary#1

Maggie

```
GENTLE DENTAL, P.C.                          PATIENT CARE FORM                    HCS  10:30  03/29/97
  Cathy A. Schmidt                                                                    75495  03/29/97

  36317-1       PATIENT        CHART #    GUARANTOR       CHART #    ACCOUNT               BALANCES   02/28/97

  PREFERRED:    Mrs. Maggie               Mr. Gary                   CSC                   CURRENT       0.00
  NAME:         Margaret Meineke          Gary L. Meineke            Code       I         ov30          0.00
  ADDRESS:      2003 NAYTOR DRIVE SE      2003 NAYTOR DRIVE SE       CREDIT OK ? Y         ov60          0.00
                CEDAR RAPIDS, IA 52403    CEDAR RAPIDS, IA 52403     LATE CHARGE?Y         ov90          0.00
  HOME PHONE:   (319) 555-1234            (319) 555-1234             DUE NOTICE  00        ov120         0.00
  WORK PHONE:   555-4322                  (319) 555-1234             NOTE DATE             PRIVATE       0.00

  REFERRED BY:  Yellow Pages    05/15/94  TOTAL                      LAST PYMT             LATE CHG      0.00
  LAST REFERRED:                          THIS PERIOD                AMOUNT      0.00      INSURANCE     0.00
  BIRTHDATE:    06/02/51
  APPOINTMENT:  No appointment scheduled                                                  TOTAL         0.00


  PERSONL CODES: Job           Orality         Source           Hobbies        RefDoc      ReferOut
                 Technician                                     Snow Skiing

=================================================== P A T I E N T   M E S S A G E S ===================================
  Recall        Watch #30 distal.                                                         HCS   03/27/97

================================================= I N S U R A N C E   I N F O R M A T I O N =============================
  SUBSCRIBER    EMPLOYER          INSURANCE CO      RENEWAL  MAX  DEDUCT  Diagn Preve Resto Perio Dentu Crown Surge Endo  O.MAX
  Gary          Rockwell          Delta Dental       1/01  1200           80    80    85    50    50    85    85    50    0
                ROCKWELL   Emergency services are covered at 100%                                            BCC  09/11/95
                           Fluoride is covered for depedent children to age 18 6 mo                          BCC  09/11/95
                           BW's are covered at 6mo                                                           BCC  09/11/95
                           Sealants are covered at 100% for dependents uder age 14                           BCC  09/11/95
                DD         Office calls are not covered,can use palliative trt. if                           JAH  12/28/91
                           applicable.                                                                       JAH  12/28/91
                           Perio scale(4345) is no longer a payable procedure.They                           BCC  06/03/96
                           will pay for 4355 PDB, but only as a pre-perio procedure.                         BCC  06/03/96
                           Debridement is to enable comprehensive perio evaluation.                          BCC  06/03/96
                           Debridement is not payable if an exam is performed first.                         BCC  06/04/96
                           For partials tooth #'s for the teeth we are replacing are                         BCC  02/06/96
                           required.                                                                         BCC  02/06/96
                           Use PROCH(1120) for age 13 and under.                                             BCC  06/03/96
                           Use PROPH(1110) for age 14 and over.                                              BCC  06/03/96
                           Documentation is required for all: Crowns, Gingivectomy,                          BCC  02/06/96
                           Gingivolplasty, Osseous surgery, root plaining and B-ups                          BCC  02/06/96
                           DD does not pay for second cleanings, the patient needs to                        BCC  06/03/96
                           be explained to that it will be their responsibility.                             BCC  06/03/96
                           Exams are not payable the same day as PMT                                         BCC  06/04/96
                CONTRACT   123456789

=================================================== F A M I L Y   M E M B E R S =======================================
  #  NAME    SEX AGE DR HY RF Lastvsit Prophy  Bitewing Panorex Dentures Relines RMAX RDED #TP NEXT APPOINTMENT   NEXT RECALL
  0 Gary     M 43 KNI CAS 6                                              1200 0  0
  1 Maggie   F 45 KNI CAS 6 11/05/02 11/05/02 04/01/02 11/01/99         1200 0  0
  Adult cleaning - _____          PSR
  Youth cleaning - _____
  Child cleaning - _____          _____  _____  _____  PAYMENT: _____

  Fluoride treatment _____        _____  _____  _____  __Cash ___Check ___MC/ VISA/ DISC/ AM EX

  Bitewing X-rays _____
  Panorex X-rays  _____
  Peri X-rays     _____

  Exam ____ Init _____
       PRV
```

Figure 1.6 Patient Care Form for Maggie

Gary's insurance information is also on the PCF. On our computer we have the major insurance companies' policies, as well as the types of insurances offered at area businesses. For instance, a large aerospace company is located just down the street from us. The company has two plans from Delta Dental, one for salaried employees and one for hourly wage earners. Both plans are listed under the aerospace company's name, where they can be added (or deleted, if need be) from a patient's chart. If the patient doesn't know his dental plan, we can easily check through his employment status.

Having the insurance information printed out is handy while chairside. No need to look in the computer to see if Gary's plan includes an adult fluoride treatment. Ellen can just glance down his form, and instantly she knows it will cover one treatment a year at 80 percent. This allows her to help the patient make a careful, informed decision on his treatment. She can say, "Gary, would you like a fluoride treatment today? Your portion of the fluoride treatment will be only three dollars out-of-pocket."

When patients know the cost, they can figure the cost/benefit analysis themselves. Dental hygienists inform them of periodontal disease, show them proper brushing and flossing, recommend plans of treatment, and discuss the benefits of fluoride. We are relaying information. It's part of our job. And often this means talking money. When we can also inform the patient of his monetary obligations, we are helping him to make informed choices.

If you have trouble talking money, remember this: When we present all data to our patients, including fees, our patients are well-informed and appreciative. If they don't know costs involved, they can't make intelligent decisions. It's a service we provide to help our patients play an active role in their dental treatment.

Quoting fees is not evil or greedy, it's informative and honest.

For example, when I take my car in for an oil change, I find out I also need a serpentine belt and my brakes are wearing. Yes, I'm distressed at the added expense. Yes, I'm trying to figure out how to pay for the brakes and school tuition. But that's okay. I know the value of my car to me—not to the mechanic or the garage owner, but to me. I'm thankful the mechanic explained the details up front including cost. It felt honest and I knew he wasn't trying to pull one over on me. Now I'm free to make the right decision for me and my bank account. It may not be the best course of action for my car, but will be the best course of action for me.

If "speaking fees" is difficult for you, then you're not alone. Many hygienists wish they didn't have to talk about money matters. However, we do not have fully socialized healthcare in the United States. Free enterprise is our way of life for the most part. Most of your patients know that dental treatment is an added expense. If they want to take care of their dental health, there is a cost involved. It's as simple as that.

By telling them of the benefits involved with a certain procedure, such as a fluoride treatment, you are helping them. Part of that information includes the fee. You are doing your patient a great service in letting him know the cost. Give him the facts and let him make up his own mind. It's true informed patients make better oral health decisions.

Ellen tells Gary the benefits of an office fluoride treatment. She lists the reasons why he should consider getting one each time he comes in for a cleaning. Then she tells him his cost. She's laid the information out for him to consider, and it's up to him to make a decision. He'll decide what he can afford.

At the bottom of Gary's PCF is an area for the hygiene assistant or hygienist to note the procedures done during today's visit, including three types of prophys, categories for a fluoride treatment, bitewings, pan, periapical x-ray, and the name of the dentist who performed the exam. If Ellen completes a periodontal debridement (PDB), she can write PDB on the line next to "adult prophy." If it's a regular cleaning, she can merely make a check on the line.

If she completes a full mouth probe, she'll note that in the computer. If Periodontal Screening and Recording (PSR) scores are within limits, she can write the numbers in the sextant boxes at the bottom of the PCF for later delivery into the computer system. Or she can relate this and other information to the hygiene assistant, who will use the PCF for notes and take it to the computer for entry. Completed PCFs are often well-worn and covered in scribbles and notes that aid in entering data into the computer. PCFs are to be used, abused, and then turned into refuse.

Cameras are easily adapted to computer systems. Intraoral cameras can aid in patient home care. They can also show cracked fillings and areas of decay, thus allowing the patient to be brought into the treatment planning process. This is not selling, this is informing. And it's vital for your patients' overall oral health.

Since the dawn of the television age, people have become much more visually-oriented. Red, inflamed marginal gingiva covered by a thin layer of plaque, or a cracked filling, present an astounding visual image. Your patient will surely take notice. Try some disclosing solution and see what your patient thinks of the mandibular lingual molar region.

Videos work nicely with computers, too. We have consent forms on video. A smiling woman named Britta, dressed to look like an assistant, carefully goes over all the bad things that can potentially happen during root canals, extractions, and crowns. (Right now our office is creating oral home care and denture home care videos to show our patients.) Wireless headsets ensure privacy and save us from boring repetition. Patients sign their consent onto a hand-held computer, similar to the package delivery company's hand-held unit.

Note that gloved hands are never used with computers in the office. In this EDO, only clean, naked hands touch a keyboard, mouse, or screen. Every office has its own system of infection control and computers. There is no right way or wrong way, as long as there is no cross-contamination.

Once Ellen completes the prophy, and Gary receives his treatment plan (Fig. 1.7), she's ready to set up his next appointment. In Gary's case, that means an "OP" (operative) appointment with the dentist and an "R6" (recall, six months) with Ellen.

She walks Gary to the computer terminal. If she hasn't entered the charges, she does so, while asking Gary to help himself to a toothbrush in a bin next to the monitor. She then checks doctor's schedule. He has an opening next week that Gary accepts.

Then she glances at her schedule six months down the road, saying, "I can see you on another Thursday at three; would that work?" Gary smiles and nods. She hands him his appointment cards, lets him know he'll receive a postcard a couple weeks before his next cleaning, and tells him she'll notify him the day before.

```
36317-0          P A T I E N T   T R E A T M E N T   P L A N
                 GENTLE DENTAL, P.C.

For:   Gary L. Meineke
       2003 NAYTOR DRIVE SE
       CEDAR RAPIDS    IA    52403

       Service Description    Prv Tooth          Fee       Insurance       Patient
Treatment Phase 1
       1st Appt. +/- 60 min.  KNI                  .00
       Crown Prep-1/2 Due     KNI LL 2nd Molar     .00
       Buildup                KNI LL 2nd Molar   99.00                       99.00
       Pin Retention          KNI LL 2nd Molar   17.00                       17.00
       Pin Retention          KNI LL 2nd Molar   17.00                       17.00

       Subtotal                                 133.00                      133.00
Treatment Phase 2
       2nd Appt. +/- 30 min.  KNI                  .00
       Crown Porcelain        KNI LL 2nd Molar  399.00                      399.00

       Subtotal                                 399.00                      399.00
Treatment Phase 3
       3rd Appt. +/- 45 min.  KNI                  .00
       Adult Cleaning         CAS                39.00                       39.00
       Fluoride Trmnt. Adult  CAS                15.00                       15.00
       Periodic Oral Exam     KNI                16.00                       16.00

       Subtotal                                  70.00                       70.00

Total:                                          602.00                      602.00
```

Gentle Dental will honor this plan for the next 3 months. After that, it will
need to be updated before it is begun. If this plan has been presented
without first having a cleaning, x-rays and exam, those procedures must be
performed before this plan can be perfected and performed.
THIS IS AN ESTIMATE ONLY.
Gentle Dental is pleased to offer 6 methods of deferred payment: MasterCard,
Visa, Discover, American Express and our own, 6 or 12 month no-interest
payment plan. All deferred plans require credit worthiness, as determined by
the finance resource.
If you are interested in the no-interest payment plan, please ask for details.

BUILD UP. Before putting a crown on a tooth, often we must replace missing
parts of the tooth like old fillings or decay. Anchor pins are placed in the
tooth and bonded plastics are used to rebuild the tooth.

CROWN PREP. To prepare for a crown we must remove the outer shell of enamel
from the tooth, which is painlessly whisked away with high speed instruments.
The sound, healthy part of the tooth is saved. It normally takes a week to
make a crown.

1/2 OF THE CROWN FEE IS DUE AT THE TIME THE CROWN PREP IS DONE.

CROWN. Crowns are precision-made thimbles of metal that fit over a tooth.
They can be silver, gold or covered with porcelain to look exactly like a
tooth. Crowns restore the tooth for many years.
Crowns must be seated within approximately 3 weeks of the prep date. If a
remake is needed, one half of the original fee will be charged.

Healthy teeth grow in healthy gums. Healthy gums can only live next to clean
teeth. That's why Gentle Dental Hygienists clean teeth three ways: 1. with
revolving cups of polishing paste; 2. with sound waves that vibrate away
debris; and 3. the old-fashioned way, by paring off debris by hand. During
cleaning, your hygienist detects disease, closely measures past destruction
and determines your personal cleaning needs. When it has been a long time
since the last cleaning--or when people rapidly accumulate tartar--one
cleaning may not do the job. Then your hygienist schedules more cleaning
appointments.

Fig. 1-7 Patient Treatment Plan

Ellen then takes Gary to the front desk where he checked in. Darlene is there with a big ol' smile. Ellen thanks him and returns to hygiene. Darlene cross-references what's on her computer screen with the scribbles on Gary's PCF. She okays the charges and prints Gary a receipt. "Your portion for today is 20 percent, or $31 dollars."

Gary pays, takes his receipt and appointment cards ("Thanks, Gary. We'll see you next week!"), and is out the door. Every aspect of Gary's visit was enhanced by the use of computers.

The Electronic Hourglass

Patience is a virtue, and a necessary commodity when dealing with computers. Then again, patience is a necessary commodity when dealing with any issue. With computers, we just need to exercise it more often.

We've come to expect instantaneous access in our society. Microwaves, remote controls, speed dials—we can hardly wait for anything. If it doesn't happen here and now, we can't wait. This is not necessarily detrimental, as technological advancement has improved our society greatly. It's difficult to remember how long it took to get up off the couch and change the channel. That was back when our televisions had dials and there were only four program choices at a time—ABC, CBS, NBC, and PBS. Now we flip through 80 channels a minute, garnering immediate gratification.

We look at computers in the same way. Think about an ATM machine. If it doesn't spit out 20s within 60 seconds, we're addled. It's a wonderful computer, that ATM machine. From a 7-Eleven on a street corner in Dallas, it reads your balance in an account in Chicago and withdraws or transfers money in less than a minute. These are truly amazing times that we live in.

Just as stunning are computers in dental offices. Files, charts, and histories appear in a flash before our eyes. Milliseconds after punching access keys, data materializes on the screen. Patient information is available, quickly and accurately. It can be collated, cross-referenced, and manipulated in seconds. We can find out in seconds how many fluoride treatments we performed last month or what our production figures were for the last quarter.

Sometimes computers don't move at lightning-fast speed. Screens don't pop up like they should, and the system seems to be dragging. Maybe there's drain on the memory because someone is running a large report, or maybe there's a system error. Whatever the cause, we just need to exert a little patience.

Patience with computers is important because when something goes wrong (and it will) we shouldn't lose our cool. Computers are nothing but machines, like a washer and dryer, a car, or a boat (read: hole in water into which money is poured). Only computers break down more often than the washer and dryer, and less often than the boat.

Things go wrong with computers and they need to be repaired, just like the autoclave, handpieces, lights, and dental chairs. It's usually more devastating because computers are our link to information. We are paralyzed without patient data. So, we can suffer terribly when computers are not working.

This is where patience is virtuous. Yes, everyone knows the computers are down. Yes, it's difficult for us to do our jobs. But we do what we can, and we know that the computers will be up and running ASAP. We're dental hygienists, and our job is hygiene. We know we aren't computer technicians who can solve the problem, so we continue with what we do best: hygiene.

The World Wide Wait

The World Wide Web is not-so-lovingly referred to as the World Wide Wait, because that's what you do. Officially, it's known as the Internet. The WWW (Wait or Web, whichever you prefer) contains all the Internet species, such as e-mail, news groups, and Internet fragments. The WWW is the way most of us use the Internet.

The WWW was developed by scientists at CERN (the European Particle Physics Laboratory in Geneva, Switzerland). It puts all things Internet under one roof, like a big warehouse. Instead of going to each boutique store to get your information, you can shop at the warehouse and get it all.

To help you shop the WWW warehouse, you can use an online service such as Compuserve, America Online (AOL), and others. Or, you can access the WWW directly through web browsing programs that are installed in newer computers.

You may have heard the expression "dot com" (".com"), when referring to an e-mail address. (E-mail stands for electronic mail.) It's the Internet's manner of categorizing you. (Fig 1.8.) An e-mail designation is nothing but an address. Your postal carrier delivers mail, referred to as snail mail, to your home address. The Internet delivers mail to your computer address.

My e-mail address is: Cathyrdh@aol.com.

Abbreviation	Affiliation
.com	business and commercial
.edu	educational institutions
.gov	governmental institutions
.mil	military installations
.net	network resources
.org	non-profit, or others

Fig. 1-8 E-mail Affiliations

My postman knows I live on Tenth Street, just as my e-mail system knows I live at aol.com. My snail mail comes to Cat Schmidt, as my e-mail comes to Cathyrdh. E-mail routings are nothing but addresses. Please feel free to e-mail me if you have suggestions or comments.

If you'd like to check out the ADHA on the World Wide Web, access:

http://www.adha.org

When hygienists go online, they will find many web sites, or web pages, devoted to dentistry. Nearly every dental school is on the web as well as some dental hygiene schools. Most major dental manufacturing companies can be located on the web and contacted there as well. The Internet, for all it's bad press regarding pornography, really offers a cornucopia of knowledge on a variety of subjects.

If you're interested in what's hot and new on the internet regarding our profession, or dentistry in general, try using a *web browser*. A web browser is a search system that will locate all references to a word, or a string of words. Simply type in a word such as "dentistry" and the browser will give you a listing of all references to dentistry. One word of caution: the less detailed your search word, the greater the number of references that will be returned to you. An entry such as "dental" will generate hundreds of options.

Other offerings for hygienists on the Internet include dental libraries, dental hygiene associations, career expansion, product information, expanded functions, continuing education, and more. There are anti-fluoride and anti-mercury groups with their own sites that we can access to learn what the "other side" is up to. Knowing your opponents' tenets can be vital to a successful debate. The wealth of information available on the Internet is nearly overwhelming. Basically, any information you require is accessible with the touch of a keyboard.

Most community colleges offer short courses to learn more about computers and the Internet. If you're interested in setting up a home computer with internet access, or if your office is becoming computerized, you may want to check into various courses offered at your community college to learn more about this expanding technology. Course work is also encouraged for anyone who wants a refresher class, or even those who have been away from computers for a few years. The knowledge gained about computers is invaluable in the workplace, as well as in everyday life.

Patience is Keystrokes

While writing this chapter on computers, my computer broke down. Not once, but twice. Like Dave Barry says, "I'm not making this up." And, surprisingly, I remained calm and collected. Computers for all their wondrous technology and assistance can be exasperating when not functioning.

My problems first started when my computer's disk drive ate a diskette. It sucked it in and wouldn't spit it back out. The drive became a black hole for disks. That's when I made a tactical error. I brought out a pair of pliers. Silly me, I thought if it wouldn't let me have my disk, I was just going to take it. Clasping the pliers tightly upon the partially ejected diskette, I yanked. Hard. Bad move.

The good news was apparent immediately. The disk was now in my hand and not wedged inside that marvel of technology, or the black hole, or whatever I called it at the time, which I'm sure I can't print here. To my credit, I was at home, not at work, where I would have been expected to act in a most professional manner, which probably means I wouldn't have used the pliers. (I would have been smarter and used an optical.)

The bad news sunk in slowly, like a Land Rover disappearing into thick quicksand. The little metal part on the disk (technical name: metal part on disk), was no longer on the disk. It was lost inside the black hole. This is terrible news for a writer, especially a writer reaching deadline with a large amount of memory stored on her computer. With the metal part obstructing the disk drive, no disk can be inserted. If no disk can be inserted, then no backup copy can be made. With no backup copy, then there's no protection in case of computer crash.

It was doubly disheartening because not only did I have to get the computer fixed, I had to make sure they protected my memory during servicing and got it done quickly, say, in less than an hour. Posthaste, I took my computer to a local repair shop, where one of the guys removed the metal part. However, he informed me the drive that reads the diskette was scratched, so it was just better to replace the whole thing. I gave the go-ahead, and within an hour I lugged my computer back out the door.

Once home, I couldn't make a backup disk. Somehow, my mouse wasn't working. No arrow, no jack. Jack is the little jack-in-the-box symbol that was an option on my mouse. He pops out of his box every time I make a certain command. He helps me keep my sense of humor. Anyway, the mouse didn't work. I checked the connection, but it was solid. I checked the cable, but it seemed intact. There was nothing for me to pull with pliers, so I called the shop again.

They said it worked fine in the shop, so this time they sent someone out to my home. He came and inspected, changed data, and tinkered with my computer through one long cup of coffee. Finally, he figured it out. With all of his technological expertise, and surrounded by computer tools and parts and disks that he had brought with him, do you know how he fixed my mouse? With a paper clip.

Yes, a simple paper clip and a pair of wire cutters did the trick. You see, a pin had dislodged from the cable connection on my computer, so he replaced it by inserting a snippet of paper clip into the corresponding female port. This completed the connection between mouse and computer, enabling them to talk with one another. He said the pin probably became worn and fell off due to my recent unhooking and rehooking the connection. He said not to touch it until I was finished with my book, and then he'd replace the male port, one with all the pins attached. Great, I said. And he didn't even charge me for the house call. Even better.

So the lesson here is that computers will break down. They will crash, they will become damaged, they will be able to be fixed with terribly expensive drives as well as paper clips. The key to working with computers is to take a "down" computer in stride. Anyone who works with computers knows that for all the good they bring, there's going to be a little hassle along the way. As dental hygienists, we're extremely lucky. Performing our jobs is not reliant upon the operation of a computer system. Computers can greatly enhance our work environment and free us to spend more time with our patients, but we are not chained to the computer. If our office computer crashes, we have all the means to continue to treat our patients with the excellent dental care we deliver.

C h a p t e r   T w o

Covering Your Assets:
Insurance and Legal Issues

"We do not have to manufacture crises in our lives; we have merely to recognize they exist."

–M. Scott Peck,
from *The Different Drum*

Ensure You're Insured

There is one item of protection that hygienists may want while at the chair in addition to a pair of gloves, a mask, and a clinic jacket. It's not a face shield, a pair of glasses, or an ultraviolet light shield. It's malpractice insurance. For hygienists who own their own businesses, such as temporary agencies or independent practices, malpractice insurance is a requirement. For the rest of us, it's a good suggestion. Yes, most hygienists are normally covered under our employer's plan, but do we require proof that he has up-to-date insurance? And just because our dentist carries malpractice insurance we can't assume we are covered

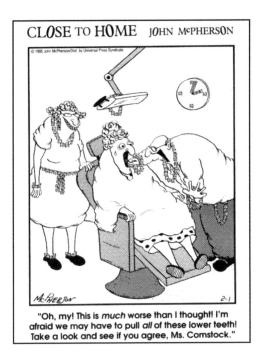

CLOSE TO HOME   JOHN McPHERSON

"Oh, my! This is *much* worse than I thought! I'm afraid we may have to pull *all* of these lower teeth! Take a look and see if you agree, Ms. Comstock."

for all possible liabilities under his plan, even as an employee.

We live in litigious times, and our safest bet is to cover our assets. It is judicious for every practicing hygienist to carry her own policy. We cannot even begin to imagine the hefty costs and emotional trauma involved in malpractice suits. We will never make enough money, ever, as dental hygienists in our lifetimes to get out of the hole a major lawsuit will dig us into. Not all people are honest and decent and good. Some may smile to our face, and then turn around and stab us in the back. We won't have even seen it coming.

Sally practiced four days a week in Dr. Loren's office. She had worked there for 10 years. Sally knew all of her patients by name and shared a great rapport with all of them. She was a loved and requested hygienist. Everything was wonderful. Or so she believed.

Dr. Loren called Sally into his office before she left for the evening. His face was ashen, his demeanor somber.

"Sally, we've just been hit with a lawsuit."

Sally gasped. She immediately felt terrible for Dr. Loren. How hard this must be for him, she thought. Her mind shot to her job. Was that selfish of her? She hoped he wouldn't have to close the practice.

"Oh, Dr. Loren, I'm so sorry for you," she said.

"That's kind of you Sally, but save some of that empathy for yourself. You've been named in the suit, as well."

You could've pushed her over with a feather.

Luckily, both Dr. Loren and Sally had separate malpractice insurance policies. They didn't have to proceed with costly court cases all on their own, and Sally had the assurance that an insurance company was looking after her needs alone, without regard to the dentist.

As happens with most lawsuits of this nature, the insurance companies settled out of court. It's usually cheaper to pay than to fight. Litigation is expensive, and people who are searching for an easy buck will take the cash in Monty's hand over door number three every time.

If you are practicing now and own your own business, or work with only your employer's malpractice insurance, look into the possibility of obtaining some of your own. Even the most perfect hygienist in the world can't compete against a patient who desires money more than morals.

The Arbitration Situation

Psst...pass it on. My dad, Schmidty, was having lunch with his attorney friend one day a few years ago. His friend was in the dumps because his firm had just been hit with a large settlement, thus staving off a professional liability lawsuit. But, he assured, Schmidty, it would never happen again.

Why? Because the firm began requiring what many national companies do now: they form an agreement with their employees, clients, or customers/patients for binding arbitration. In other words, everyone involved gives up their right to sue.

Is this legal? Usually. You may have signed one yourself. If you've had dealings with moving lines, auto agencies, attorneys, health-care providers, insurance companies, unions, banks, or brokerage firms, you may have given away your right to sue by signing an arbitration agreement. It's legal and it's fair.

A binding arbitration agreement states that if there is a dispute, the matter will not be taken to court, but will be resolved through an impartial expert. This expert understands both the subject matter and the arbitration process. One obtains the expert through the American Arbitration Association (AAA).

The AAA is an administrative organization that handles 60,000 claims a year, without prejudice. For a filing fee of around $500 (usually, both parties equally share the cost), they will handle the arbitration process. The process is one that is timely and just. After the dispute has been filed with AAA and the fee paid, both parties receive a list of potential arbitrators and their credentials. Each party then ranks the arbitrators according to preference. After one has been chosen by AAA, as determined by each party's liking, the hearing date and time are selected. No jury, no trial, no lengthy court battles or steep lawyers' fees. It's reasonable, fair and quick.

Both parties really win in this situation because it does save on costs and tension. Frivolous filing is usually nonexistent, as someone searching for quick cash is not going to fork out $250 to file. Also, these people seeking quick bucks have no chance of getting an "out-of-court settlement," which is what most lawsuit filers obtain. Attorneys know this. That's why there are so many lawsuits filed against practitioners by lawyers on contingency. Even if the practitioner is 100 percent in the right, the insurance company will still settle out of court. The only reason? It's cheaper to settle than to fight.

Another benefit of arbitration is that there are no juries to manipulate. A woman rendered edentulous by foregoing dental treatment (periodontal disease) immediately earns the empathy of a jury. Even if the practitioner did nothing to cause this condition, the jury feels sorry for the woman who lost her all her teeth, and will be swayed in her favor. The jury figures the practitioner has insurance, and since insurance is going to pay anyway, why not give something to this poor woman? It's odd that when the money is coming out of the pocket of a large corporation, or from an insurance policy, some people can see unmerited payment as innocuous. Unjustified payouts by insurance companies resulting from chimerical lawsuits account for increased insurance premiums for everyone.

An insurance company would never go to trial with a case like the edentulous woman. It would be much better to settle beforehand. The innocent practitioner, who could be any one of us, is scarred for life. Innocence is no guarantee of justice in court trials because juries base their decisions on both fact and emotion. Usually emotion wins. And which side has more support, the minimum-wage-earning edentulous woman or the hygienist who makes $25 an hour and has insurance? I'm not an astrophysicist, but methinks the edentulous woman's going to get a bundle.

If you think by foregoing insurance you'll offset any court problems, please rethink that logic. If you have no insurance, and there is a judgment against you personally, the court can garnish your wages for life, take away your house, car, or any other property you own, or have you take out a loan to pay the sum requested. It may haunt you the rest of your life. Malpractice insurance could be beneficial. I must stress that malpractice insurance is not a guarantee—nothing ever is—but it can help if you are sued and you are in the right.

Every single patient in our office, whether in for a cleaning or a tooth extraction, has signed this binding arbitration agreement:

"I agree that any dispute about the reasonableness of computation of fees, or any claim of negligent or intentional acts or omissions in the rendering of professional services, either in this instance or in any other treatment rendered by staff in this office, shall be submitted to binding arbitration under Chapter 579A of the Code of Iowa (1993). It is understood by both doctors and patient that by agreeing to submit all claims or assertions that either the patient or doctor may have against the other arising out of this agreement, patient and doctor have given up their right to a jury or court trial."[2]

Does it work for us? It hasn't been tested yet by court action. Will it work in your state? It depends upon the laws of your state. Many national companies have used binding arbitration for years, and more are joining every day. The movement is toward binding arbitration and away from personal lawsuits. Binding arbitration appears to be the panacea for the deluge of spurious lawsuits swamping our court system.

When you share this information with your employer, inform him that he must check with his lawyer and his professional liability insurance carrier for their opinions and permissions. Since laws differ from state to state, legal counsel is vital. I cannot stress this enough.

For more information contact:

American Arbitration Association
1101 Walnut Street, Suite 903
Kansas City, MO 64106-2110
(816) 471-5264

Documentation

As dental hygienists, our best defense against the nasties in the world is our own documentation. Document, document, document, then document some more should be our credo. And this does not just apply to patient care. Documentation within the workplace regarding employers and co-workers can be our safety net. Documenting actions, conversations, and remarks can aid us in an employment dispute, a co-worker tangle, or a patient complaint (against us). Proper notation can be career-saving.

Documentation can be as simple as jotting down a few paragraphs regarding a specific incident and noting the date and time. Experts reccomend keeping it on file for at least seven years, although it may seem antiquated after only a few months. Really, the amount of time one keeps this information depends on the incident, and if legal action could ever result. Obviously, if there would be need in the future for such information from a legal standpoint, it's better to keep it filed away for a longer duration of time.

Documentation also can be as formal as typing a report of an incident and having the involved parties sign the description along with a notary signature. A document such as this should remain in the files for a number of years. If the incident requires this type of documentation, it would be wise to seek advice from a trusted friend, colleague, or lawyer. If you have been wronged, or feel you might be a scapegoat in an office incident, do not hesitate to seek legal counsel to discuss your options and to learn how to behave from that point forward. Many employees lose their chance at a fair settlement because of inappropriate responses to accusations. Even talking to a trusted mentor can help walk you through the anger, so that you do not run the risk of flying off the handle.

If this piece of advice sounds hypocritical after lauding the ability of arbitration, it's not. Documentation will help you in an arbitration dispute, as well as a lawsuit. Arbitration is impartial, and you will have your chance to explain your side to the professional mediator. Just because you have signed an arbitration agreement doesn't mean you cannot seek legal counsel. Simply be prepared for the out-of-pocket expenses incurred with counsel.

Documenting inappropriate acts of co-workers, when your employer has turned a deaf ear to your calls of "foul," will demonstrate your distance from the issue. If you feel that maybe down the road you will get blamed for actions by a co-worker, make copious notes regarding each incident. An exemplary idea is to write a paragraph or two about the circumstance as soon as possible afterwards. Then, a day later, review your notes, rewriting if necessary to dispel any anger or undue emotion. Make sure your notes appear unbiased so that they will be viewed as factual by neutral parties. Your notes should read like a newspaper account of the incident. When in doubt, answer the key questions of journalism: what, who, where, and when. Then complete your report with your signature and the date, and keep it in a safe place.

For disputes with your employer that have not been resolved through discussion directly with your boss, you may want to consider obtaining documentation from other sources, such as patients and co-workers. This must be done with utmost discretion and respect for all parties considered: patient, co-worker, employer, and yourself. To drag others into our fights is morally and ethically irresponsible behavior. If a co-worker or a patient confronts us with an issue identical or similar to our dispute, proceeding with documentation could be justified. Seeking these individuals outright to aid our cause is dangerous and foolish, as we could end up on the receiving end of a reprimand or worse.

As dental hygienists, we all know that documenting patient interaction chairside is vital to our continued success. We need to remember that whatever oddity arises in the appointment must be written in the ledger notes, as well as the mundane facts of a routine prophy. If there are any special items to consider, or if a procedure was completed, or not performed, then note-taking is required. Should a special circumstance occur, a debate could surface on whether to transcribe the event or not. Remember: when in doubt, document.

Documentation is key to our protection in dental hygiene. If your writing skills are minimal, do not fret as documentation does not need to be written in proper English with correct punctuation. The key to successful documentation is to ensure that the main point is understood. A good notation of events does not concentrate on the setup but shoots straight for the heart of the matter. Background information can be added later, if it's necessary. Stick to the facts in your notation regarding the actual event or conversation, and you've got yourself a winner.

Insurance Assurance

The original disco era was in its infancy when insurance first materialized in dentistry. Since the 1970s, dental insurance has increased the need for dentists and hygienists. Thanks to dental insurance more people than ever are seeking the services we provide. Dental insurance keeps our recall patients towing the line.

New patients come in after years away from a dental chair saying: "I would have come sooner, but I didn't have dental insurance." Insurance has become nearly a prerequisite to dental visits. If insurance isn't going to help pay, they reason, then they can't afford an appointment. This is a tragic misconception in the public sector, and one reason why only 50 percent of all Americans seek dental care. Insurance should not be a necessity before people obtain dental treatment, but sadly economics plays a role.

It is this very situation where our job to educate the public comes into play. We need to inform the public about the real expense of missed dental recalls, both monetarily (in the cost of extra work for root canals and root planing) and physically (in the damage done by caries and periodontal disease). Insurance or not, missed recalls add up to enormous losses for our patients.

As more employers offer dental insurance as a benefit of employment, more people will be able to afford dental care. With an increase in patients seeking dental treatment, and with insurance companies realizing the benefits of preventive dentistry, the role and function of hygienists in dental care delivery will expand. This will be seen through various forms of insurance, most notably managed-care (see section on managed-care in this chapter).

Insurance can often dictate or direct our mode of treatment, which is not as bad as it sounds. Insurance can be hygiene-friendly. When dealing with a patient who has insurance, there are three important steps to follow.

Step 1. Design the course of treatment without consulting the insurance. Base your decisions on the patient needs alone and devise a treatment plan listing the best courses of action.

Step 2. Cross-refer your treatment plan with what the insurance allows to see if insurance covers the treatment as designed. If needed, can it be altered to give the maximum benefit to both the patient's health and his checkbook? Can a different ADA code be used so that the insurance will allow it, and it will perform the same function as your original estimation?

Step 3. Propose the revised treatment plan to the patient or both your version and the insurance-altered version. Explain your reasoning on which course the patient should take. In preparing treatment choices, we must be careful not to overwhelm the patient, but simply provide different options of dental care. Our judgment and instincts should be used with every case.

The second step is performed as a benefit for the patient. If we aren't compromising patient health, then why not give them an option? Hygienists do this every time we offer fluoride. Many insurance companies do not pay for fluoride benefits for adults. This, we know to be ludicrous. But if our patients refuse fluoride unless it's covered, then our patients go without a fluoride treatment. That's when the second step comes into play.

Those people whose insurance companies do not pay for fluoride treatment have insurance prescription cards. These cards let them have prescriptions at very low rates. Prescriptions include fluoride gel for home use. Bingo. The patient refused a $15 dollar office fluoride treatment. However, he can travel to his pharmacy and get a prescription of Prevident 5000 for five bucks. Thanks to our clever thinking, he gets the fluoride he needs.

A patient comes in who doesn't present with periodontal pocketing, but has what we'd call a "grunge mouth." So, Step 1: you decide that she could really stand a couple of prophys to get her back on track. Step 2, you check her insurance. It will cover two cleanings in a 12-month period. Step 3: you tell the patient her insurance will pay at 80 percent for both prophys (and bitewings and exam), but when she comes in for her six-month recall, she'll have to pay for it herself. Then, if she stays on a six-month recall, the insurance will pay at 80 percent for each prophy.

Great. The patient's happy because she's using her insurance and you're happy because she gets the treatment you know she needs. It's a win-win situation when a patient's insurance can be used to afford them the dental care they deserve.

Know the Code

Dental insurance is tricky business. As dental hygienists, even if we don't directly file claims or handle charges, we must understand insurance codes. It's important for us to know these codes so we can charge for the correct procedures.

I won't spend the time going over codes here. The world of codes is ever-changing—sometimes daily. Remember when we used 4345? Now it's practically nonexistent. The insurance companies felt we overused the code, and now refuse to pay it. This is typical behavior for insurance companies regarding codes. If we actually use them, they are taken away from us. In our office we can still use the 4345 code on Title XIX patients, because it's the only way to allow them to have multiple cleanings (first and second pros) if they don't present with criteria for root planing.

We need to understand the American Dental Association (ADA) codes so we can properly treat our patients to the best utilization of their insurance. We benefit, the patient benefits, and even the insurance company benefits. Carol Tekavec, RDH, is an expert on insurance. She has authored books on the subject and written columns in various publications, including *Dental Economics*. She is an excellent resource for continued understanding of the complexity of dental codes.

We benefit from knowing the latest information on dental codes, because our patients will more easily accept treatment if the out-of-pocket expense is not high. When we make it cost-effective for the patient, the patient takes care of his/her oral needs. Therefore we more easily continue to perform our job by meeting our patients' hygiene needs.

Patients benefit because they obtain maximum use of their insurance. They feel the money committed to insurance should be put to use. If not, why have the insurance? Most want their oral needs to be met, but they want insurance to pay its fair share.

Insurance companies benefit from this arrangement because patients who do not care for their teeth usually have greater oral needs later. A regular recall cleaning schedule now is a lot cheaper than root planing and perio maintenance years from now. This saves the insurance company time and money by cutting down on their workforce for extensive filing and foregoing payout for expensive procedures.

Knowledge of codes is also important in saving your license. That story about the hygienist losing her license because her dentist filed periodontal scalings for pedo prophys is absolutely true. It really happened. And if it can happen to her, it can happen to you.

Learn the codes and know what your dentist is filing. It's your right to see what codes he has filed for procedures you have performed. Use your ledger notes liberally. As added protection, when you've done a regular six-month recall prophy, write "1110," the ADA code for such a cleaning, on the ledger.

At our office, the ADA code automatically accompanies our explosion code in the computer. If we type in "A" for adult prophy, "1110" will come up as the completed procedure. Since we file claims electronically, whatever we enter becomes the submitted code. It's up to each hygienist and assistant to ensure correct code entry.

In learning the codes we're not only helping serve our patients with better hygiene, but we're also saving our fannies. No dental board is going to accept the excuse of ignorance from a professional dental hygienist. They're smarter than that, and so are we.

Patient Payment Options

There are three ways a patient may pay for dental services: fee for service, third-party lenders, and third-party prepayment plans.

Fee for service is a two-party arrangement where a fee is established and then paid for directly by the recipient. A dentist will determine that $45 is fair for a prophy, charge this to his patient, and then the patient pays that amount per cleaning. Payment is expected the day services are rendered.

Lender agreements for payment of dental services can be arranged by each practice. For instance, in our office we offer a no-interest payment plan with approved credit. The patient applies for the loan (through a financing company) in our office and we file for him. We receive 90 percent of the patient's loan from the loan company, up front, as payment in full for dental treatment. The patient then pays the loan company directly, which keeps 10 percent of the loan as their profit. It's a practical arrangement for patients with extensive treatment plans and no insurance.

The third type of payment is through third parties with prepayment plans. That third party can be an insurance company or an employer. Dentists and patients are the first and second parties, while the insurance company would be considered the third party. The third party processes and pays claims made by the dentist for the patient. These third party plans are beneficial because they cover groups of people, not individuals. The financial burden lies upon the group. Some individuals will have no dental needs, most will have few dental needs, and a handful will have many dental needs. The economics work well for the insurance company.

Remuneration for prepayment plans is done by the usual, customary, and reasonable (UCR) fee. The UCR fee is based upon the amount that most dentists in a geographical area charge for a particular service. For instance, if 90 percent of general dentists in Plano, Texas, charge $45 for a prophy, then $45 will be considered the UCR fee for Plano general practitioners.

There are many prepayment plans. Some may include commercial insurance companies, health service corporations (dental benefits as part of health-care benefits), dental service corporations (Delta Dental, et. al.), managed-care organizations, and capitation plans. All of these are third-party payment plans.

As dental hygienists, we need to stay current with the constant changes in dental insurance. Part of our being professionals is that we research and investigate the diverse payment plans open to the public. In understanding our patients' payment options, we can better serve them and provide for their dental needs.

Managed-care Managed

Prevention is the key word for managed-care organizations and that's why managed-care and dental hygiene should be a match made in heaven. The primary focus of insurance coverage is preventive treatment. Managed-care programs are designed to meet the needs of the majority, not the individual as with traditional systems. managed-care organizations focus on a population average.

The emphasis for managed-care insurance is cost-effective treatment for both the insured and the company. Managed-care banks on keeping the population as a whole healthy through preventive measures, thereby preventing sickness and costly procedures. It pays for preventive services, hoping that few in the population base will get sick. Fewer illnesses result in lower final costs to the company. Healthy individuals do not need expensive treatment.

There are six major types of managed-care organizations:

1.EPO: Exclusive provider organization.
2.HMO: Health maintainence organization.
3.IPA: Independent practice organization
4.PHO: Physician-hospital organization.
5.POS: Point-of-service plan.
6.PPO: Preferred-provider organization.

EPO: Exclusive provider organization.
The EPO is used by employers to keep costs down while providing their employees with an insurance program. The employer will contract with a provider for services at a reduced-fee rate. The insured must use only providers and clinics that have agreed to this plan.

HMO: Health maintenance organization.
The HMO is probably the most widely-known of the managed-care organizations. A prepayment for services is expected before the patient is seen for treatment. The patient chooses from a network of specified providers or a group practice owned by the HMO. Payment is made through capitation (set amount paid yearly or monthly) to the practice.

IPA: Individual practice association.

Sixty-five percent of HMOs are IPAs. IPAs are groups of providers that negotiate with HMOs. They contract with HMOs yet retain their autonomy. These providers will be reimbursed by capitation or fee for service.

PHO: Physician-hospital organization.

PHOs consist of physicians and hospitals. This organization then contracts with HMOs and other managed-care organizations to provide services in a managed-care manner.

POS: Point-of-service plan.

POS affords the patient a choice of using either a PPO or a compensation plan. The patient has a broader range of choice as far as choosing a provider but the reimbursement may be diminished.

PPO: Preferred provider organization.

PPOs are created when insurance companies contract with providers. There is a fee schedule established for the provider and the patient must pay a portion of the fee at the time services are rendered.

Managed-care has its foot in the dental office door. It looks to be moving in, whether dentistry accepts it or not. Managed-care is cost-effective for at least three of the four entities involved: patient, patient's employer, and the insurance company. However, most dentists are not fond of managed-care.

Why not? The ADA frets that managed-care organizations give the patient a reduced fee at the dentist's expense. Some dentists feel that the plan exerts too much control over acceptable modes of treatment. Some worry about diminished quality of service for the patient. Still other dentists fear that dental offices will turn into "dental mills," or a term that we're familiar with, "prophy mills." The ADA supports fee-for-service dental care over managed-care dentistry.

One of the benefits of managed-care to dental hygiene is that it is prevention-oriented, just like hygiene. We understand the need for preventive therapy and the foundation of managed-care is prevention. It seems that managed-care and dental hygiene should go hand-in-hand. As empathetic health-care practitioners we appreciate the fact that

managed-care provides our patients with access to cost-effective preventive dentistry. With greater access to dental benefits through managed-care insurance systems, it is anticipated that more people will
seek preventive dental care provided by dental hygienists.

The American Dental Hygienists' Association (ADHA) believes
managed-care insurance in dentistry is here to stay and that prudent
behavior dictates its acceptance. Simply wishing away managed-care is
unrealistic, believes the ADHA, so why not accept the changes in our
profession so we can more astutely deal with insurance realities? As the
saying goes: Denial is not a river in Egypt. The ADA appears to be in
denial.

The ADHA does not endorse all managed-care plans, but the organization does believe that managed-care will provide greater access to
preventive dentistry for the general public and broader career opportunities for dental hygienists. In a press kit released by the ADHA regarding managed-care, the organization states:

*"Managed-care provides a framework in which to maximize and
appropriately recognize the role of dental hygienists. Managed-care and
dental hygiene naturally complement one another because both emphasize
prevention and cost-effectiveness. ADHA looks forward to a future in which
Americans can easily and affordably access the quality, cost-effective oral
health services provided by dental hygienists."*

If our goal as dental hygienists is to provide the highest quality of
dental hygiene care to the general public and to promote preventive
measures of oral health care, then managed-care could aid us in the
attainment of that goal.

On the flip side, a reduction in fees directly related to the managed-
care model may indirectly affect the dental hygienist through loss of
wages, production figures, and/or benefits. The math is easy to understand: if our employers make less, the office makes less, and we don't
get raises. If our employers are financially strong, they'll be able to provide us with the type of compensation to which we are entitled.

**Whether we like it or not, we are tied to the office profit
margin and we have to learn to accept that.**

Dr. Richard Simms, DDS, MS, stated in an article in *Dental Economics*[3] that no practitioner, whether dentist or dental hygienist, should willingly accept a 50-percent reduction in income that accompanies managed-care treatment. A 50-percent reduction in income for hygienists would correlate to income levels of the early 1980s. He also notes that if managed-care companies are so eager to save money, why would they not be just as eager to see auxiliary personnel performing the duties of dental hygienists? They may also push for legislative changes in auxiliary duties. Remember, it takes money to fight for changes in laws and managed-care organizations have plenty of money for these battles. These are all valid points for hygienists to consider when contemplating the benefits of managed-care.

The ADA vehemently opposes managed-care and has issued an opinion against the ADHA for supporting it. Some are quick to point out that the ADA's position results from both political and economic concerns. Most certainly the ADA's position has such motivation, but that's also true for the ADHA's side in the battle. All debate regarding such explosive issues is inherently politically and financially loaded. Each organization battles for causes benefiting its own profession and membership base (members = funding, ye old "money-talks" mentality). Our job as intelligent hygienists is to sift through the chaff to understand the true issue.

A scenario worth considering is that in practices where both fee-for-service and capitation patients exist, the fee-for-service patients may end up picking up the slack. If managed-care cannot properly compensate the dental office for its members, then fee-for-service patients would have to foot the bill by paying higher fees for each service rendered.

Some dentists and dental hygienists have voiced their concerns over procedural guidelines and tight scheduling pressures that accompany managed-care. A managed-care patient can become to be seen as a non-productive patient, as a problem and not a solution. This is the antithesis to the ADHA's wishes for access to preventive care treatment for many people. If these patients become burdens, preventive care will take on a whole new meaning. Read: prophy mill.

Another problem to managed-care is that a practitioner's judgments could be taking a back seat to profitability. If the dentist desires full-mouth root planing and a crown and the company negates the diagnosis, opting instead for two scales and four-surface amalgam, who benefits? Certainly not the patient, who receives below-par treatment. Definitely not the dental practice, which receives far less compensation for treatment. The managed-care insurance organization benefits. Its profits increase, while dental offices are run out of business due to lack of profit. Patients are left with substandard treatments and the feeling that they may not be getting what they've been promised. And hygienists? Perhaps the only route left would be independent practices for dental hygienists—if their practices can survive on the lower managed-care fees.

If you're in a typical practice, you probably experience a fee-for-service environment. Perhaps you work in a managed-care setting or maybe you have a mixture of insurance plans. Whatever your current position, it's in your best interest to do a little investigating and research on your own to determine your feelings about managed-care and its effects on the future of hygiene and, most importantly, your own future. Managed-care is a hot issue and it's in our best interest as hygienists to understand both the ADA's viewpoint as well as the ADHA's position on the subject. When we blindly accept a viewpoint handed to us by a group or organization, we rob ourselves of self-discovery and a chance to use our intellect. There's something wasteful and empty about a mind unused.

Direct Reimbursement

Direct reimbursement plans differ from other types of dental payment plans. Why? Because direct reimbursement (DR) does not involve insurance companies.

Direct reimbursement is just what its name indicates: the employee is directly reimbursed from the employer for dental expenses. Since there are no insurance companies involved, treatment is left in the hands of the provider, where dental treatment should be. Insurance companies do not have a say in the treatment to be performed. There are no claims to file, forms to fill out, or pre-authorization to be obtained. The dentist provides treatment and the patient pays for services and is reimbursed by his employer.

According to Roger S. Schultz, CLU in *Dental Economics*, March 1996, a typical DR plan would look something like this:

Patient portion	Employer portion
First $100 in expenses:	100 percent of fees.
Next $100 in expenses:	70 percent of fees.
Next $1660 in expenses:	50 percent of fees.

The employer pays up to $1,000 per family member.

There are two major problems with DR. One is that no one is promoting it as a viable alternative for large corporations seeking dental plans. Since brokers only obtain commissions from insurance companies and have no financial stake in DR, it is unlikely they will suggest it to their clients. Employers cannot obtain for their employees something they've never heard of. Since no broker is going to promote this plan, employers will remain in the dark unless the dental profession decides to take on the cause.

Second, companies that offer DR to their employees expect dental offices to bill patients for services and not accept payment directly following treatment. As we know, the surest way to prevent a collections hassle is to enforce the sign that reads: "Payment is expected at the time services are rendered." This is vital to a smoothly running practice. Proponents of DR claim that billing patients gives them time to receive payment from their employer. Thus, they'll have the money when the dental bill arrives. In theory this sounds spectacular. The patient receives money from the employer and sends it off to the dentist. However, those of us who are not lost in a cloud of Pollyanna perfume know where the reimbursed money goes once the check arrives in the mail—and it's not back to the dental office.

Social Insurance

In our office we refer to the Title XIX payment method as insurance. In doing so, we benefit the patient as well as other patients in the office who might hear our words. Insurance has a less-inflammatory ring to it than the terms welfare, Medicaid, or Title XIX. It doesn't matter to us which word is used, but it matters a lot to the patients on Title XIX and to the other patients within earshot.

Not every office accepts Title XIX. Some accept a limited amount of welfare patients. Maybe you work with Title XIX. Maybe you're wondering who these people are. Title XIX recipients are usually recipients of other forms of government assistance. Some may be disabled (physically or mentally), blind, or without work. Some may earn income below the poverty line. Oftentimes they are children of lower-income families. Whoever they may be, they're patients and their dental needs should be met.

It's easy to understand why dentists do not want to service Title XIX patients. A large percentage of the patients in our office are Title XIX and we've learned firsthand that these patients have special considerations that must be understood if a practice is going to treat them.

Here's a list of considerations associated with Title XIX patients:

1. These people can have numerous broken or failed appointments.
2. They usually have special needs, like intensive periodontal disease or rampant decay.
3. Compensation from the state for dental treatment is usually well below UCR.
4. The office must allot more time for appointments for the physically or mentally challenged.

In short, Title XIX recipients could be seen as burdensome patients, especially to smaller practices. It can also be very fulfilling to provide dental treatment for patients who cannot afford it or who are handicapped in some manner. The decision on whether or not to see Title XIX patients comes down to where our responsibilities lie as health-care deliverers. We entered the dental profession to provide oral hygiene care to people—all people, without bias. It's our duty as dental hygienists to see that all people have access to excellent dental care.

In 1950 my father entered dental school. A year later, my sister, Cyd, was born at the University of Iowa hospital. The state paid for my sister's birth because my father couldn't afford it. My parents were broke, and my father worked as much he could while attending dental school full-time. My father is a proud man and leaning on others during this hard time was difficult for him. He vowed then and there that he would repay the debt of my sister's birth somehow.

That's why today, if you call our office and say that you have no money and a toothache, or that you are on Title XIX, you will be given an appointment.

Chapter Three

Infection Protection:
OSHA Comes Calling

"Nothing is so much to be feared as fear."

—Henry David Thoreau
from *Journal*, September 7, 1851

Uncle Sam as Watch Dog

The Occupational Safety and Health Administration (OSHA) is a federal agency designed to protect workers from unsafe work practices. Formed in 1970, it regulates all industries in the United States. OSHA investigates, inspects, and controls all employee job functions from welder to dental hygienist.

OSHA is designed for you, the employee, the worker who may be exposed to unnecessary hazards in the workplace. It's your safety net, to guard you from harm. OSHA is the government's way of saying, "Hey, we care. We don't want you to be hurt trying to make a decent living. So, we're going to issue some rules for your employer to follow that will protect you while you work."

OSHA protects you, the employee!

OSHA investigates, controls, and monitors all types of businesses, from video store chains to dental offices. Any company that employs five or more employees or any healthcare facility where workers are exposed to biohazardous substances must follow OSHA rules. This includes dental offices, as workers there handle blood and other potentially infectious materials (BOPIM). Everyone in the dental office must comply with OSHA's Bloodborne Pathogen (BBP) standard.

When OSHA's BBP standard became effective on July 6, 1992, the profession of dentistry went into a panic. Dental offices were accordingly inspected and fined tens of thousands of dollars for noncompliance. No one, not even OSHA, truly understood the underlying effect the BBP standard would have on dentistry.

A True Story

In May of 1992, I started work in my father's dental practice. Since I moved back to the Midwest from the East, I needed to take another set of dental hygiene boards. While waiting for the results of those boards, my father put me in charge of the OSHA program for his office of 30 employees.

One has to remember that the atmosphere at the time was rather hot. OSHA was a volatile subject for both dentists and employees. The nation was in a panic over the human immunodeficiency virus (HIV) scare and the profession of dentistry found itself thrust under a microscope. Rumors abounded and misinformation about the spread of HIV and other pathogens was commonplace.

News shows on television fueled the flames. They produced inflammatory stories exposing the dangers of blood in dental handpieces, instruments, and chairs. They frightened people into thinking that merely visiting the dentist was a death sentence. At least one patient a day in our office wanted to see our sterilizing techniques, firsthand. The public was scared and so were we. Everyone had an opinion on the proper method of implementing the OSHA BBP standard. We heard a report of one dentist receiving a fine for using Lysol as an operatory disinfectant. Another was cited for having a Coke can next to the autoclave. The atmosphere at the time was pure chaos.

Dentists were scrambling to comply yet trusting no one source. Hygienists and assistants begged for information, policy changes, and safety. No one was sure of the proper method of protection. Everyone wanted it, but the BBP standard was extensive and didn't take into account the complexity and diversity of the delivery of dentistry.

Then there were the cross-contamination questions. Since OSHA is a governmental body set up to protect workers, it has no jurisdiction over patient protection. According to OSHA, as long as the worker is safe, everything is peachy-keen. OSHA can't cite offices for failing to protect the patient from BBP. To this day, the public has no grasp of that. They still believe these governmental regulations protect them when, in fact, they only really protect the dental office employee.

The times were strange and frustrating. Over-compliance was a trait common in some offices. One dentist had his hygienist dressed head to toe in scrubs (yes, a hat and shoe coverings) along with goggles, a mask and a face shield. She looked prepared to perform open heart surgery. No wonder the public was scared.

Inspections from OSHA were the public and employee buffer at the time. The strong arm of government offered an appearance of protection. This left everyone in dentistry on edge. A fine of tens of thousands of dollars could shut down a small business in a heartbeat. No one knew when OSHA would strike an office and no one was ever prepared when it did.

Teamwork

In implementing a safe work environment for 30 employees, I realized right away that I needed help. But since everyone was a novice at implementing the BBP standard in dental offices, there were no experts to call in. Everyone was a first-timer. That's when the obvious hit me like a load of bricks. There are 30 people in this office and if two heads are better than one, surely 30 should be stupendous. I was right.

I broke down the specifics for each area of the office as stated in the BBP and every employee had input into its implementation. We dissected the office into little bits, then smaller bits, until we had exact procedures and exact safety responses.

Since I had the time, the desk, and the computer, I concentrated on documentation, including forms, reports and control plans. Others in the office stepped in to help with various areas of the office that were unfamiliar to me.

I had never assisted before and so long-time assistants like Debbie and others helped with deciding which protective measures to take for different procedures. Jenny was in charge of our sterilization area and whipped that into shape in no time.

(When we moved into our new office in the winter of 1994, Pam, now in charge of sterilization, designed an area from scratch that would be both efficient to tasks and conforming to OSHA. She and Diana ensure our instruments are sterile and ready every single hour of the working day. Our new office was designed with OSHA in mind and works quite well for our present needs.)

But our old office had been converted from an early twentieth-century house. To conform to the BBP standard, we had to consider the arrangement of our office at the time, which was difficult work.

The old house was great, but cramped. The front room was designed to look just like a living room. A long narrow hallway passed by the front desk and led back to the main operatory. Two rooms leading from the hallway were a hygiene room and the x-ray room. Farther back was the doctor's office, the sterilization area and the operatory.

The office had 11 chairs in all. One in x-ray, two in hygiene, and eight in the operatory. Operatory chairs were lined up four on each side facing a little window that promised relief from claustrophobia. Privacy walls separated each chair. So, this was the problem: where exactly was the operatory? Was it confined to the space around the chair? Or did it encompass the entire room of eight chairs? And how did the hygiene room fit into the picture?

These questions and more had us baffled. Perhaps today they look rather silly and easy to answer but back then things were different. We had never pondered these issues—no dental office had—at least not until the spring of 1992.

In fact, many topics arose that we hadn't expected. One doctor refused to wear gloves. He insisted that he had gone without them for umpteen years at the chair, and he wasn't about to start. He converted. Assistants who had begged for clinic jackets to protect their clothing from splatter wore the jackets open and unbuttoned. They converted, too.

We hadn't expected the inconveniences that accompanied compliance. All the changes to routine were annoying and, at first, seemed to get in the way of dentistry. Back then the changes were overwhelming. New procedures, new rules were tough to follow. Old habits die hard, and some employees working in our office had been in dentistry for more than a decade, so change for them was toughest. It's difficult to change ingrained habits. With the advent of these new rules and regulations—for everyone, not just my office—the delivery of dentistry would never be the same.

At a couple days past the July 1992 deadline, we had barely had time to adapt to all the new changes in rules, when...

OSHA Knocks!

My dad, Schmidty, buzzed me from his office. "Cat, there's a man here from OSHA."

My heart skipped a beat. OSHA? Here? I can't say I was totally surprised. An office as large as ours attracts attention. From lawsuits (people looking for easy income) to OSHA, we're a natural choice. I figured long ago that OSHA would want to make an example of us.

Since everyone in the office was involved in the OSHA process, we had already discussed the prospect of an OSHA inspection. Actually, we knew it would happen. We just didn't know it would occur only days after the BBP standard became effective.

"I'll be right down," I answered.

On my way down the stairs I felt adrenaline rush through my veins. Fight or flight, I thought as I passed the employee entrance. This was the real thing.

As the exposure control manager for the office, I was officially in charge of the OSHA program. This was the technical truth, despite the fact everybody in the office contributed to its implementation. However, I suppose the responsibility rested on my shoulders and our program was about to be tested.

"You have been charged with five alleged safety or health hazards," said the pleasant-looking young man whose name was Jerry. "Would you like me to procure a search warrant?"

Schmidty immediately declined. That's rule number one; the inspector can get a search warrant easily enough but it'll take time and he might get irritated. Accept the situation and don't upset the nice OSHA man.

The nice OSHA man then proceeded to show us the charges. They were filed on July 7, 1992, in Des Moines, Iowa (a two-hour drive from our office in Cedar Rapids), exactly one day after the BBP standard went into effect.

They read as follows (taken verbatim from the complaint form):

HEALTH

1. The lab's pumus (*sic*) pan is used all day long and does not get cleaned at the end of the day. It hasn't been cleaned in the last month.

2. Handpieces are only autoclaved if they have blood on them.

3. Doctor only wears gloves when doing surgery. Other employees wear face shields, but are not allowed to wear face masks or lab coats because the doctor does not want the patients to feel as if they are in a dental office. He also feels that protective equipment is not necessary.

4. Coffee pot and cups for staffers is (*sic*) located in sterile lab.

SAFETY

1. Lab downstairs (dentures, crowns, etc.) has only one exit. The windows would be very hard to get out (*sic*).

There they were, in black and white. The "employee" box below was checked indicating that the complainant was an employee of the office. For me that was the most disheartening thing to see. We had all worked so closely and for so long to achieve OSHA compliance.

But it was the employee's right to complain to OSHA, and I never harbor bad feelings about it. It's your right to file a complaint, too, if you believe your employer has created an unsafe work environment. As long as you brought it to her attention, and she refused to comply with the rules, then OSHA is your safety net. When your employer refuses to change what you absolutely know to be a violation, then it's time to call OSHA.

However, make sure the hazard is a true violation and not a communication problem between you and your employer. Sometimes just opening a dialogue with your employer will lead to a better understanding of each other's positions. Your best bet is to know the law. It will help you determine true hazards in your workplace.

Let's say you find a violation in your office, you've pointed it out to your employer, and her answer is, "It's no big deal. Everybody does it." You feel that this hazard compromises your safety at work. What do you do? This is when you call OSHA for advice. Should you report it? OSHA can help you decide your next action.

You can find OSHA listed in the government pages in the phone book. Usually the agency will be located in a state's capital city. When you call you will be asked a series of questions about your employer and the alleged hazard. What you say is protected by law. You have a right to confidentiality so that your employer never may know that you called OSHA.

The employee who turned in our office for the alleged hazards opted for confidentiality. She had also checked the box that claimed she had approached the employer regarding the alleged hazards. This was not true. She spoke with neither me nor Schmidty regarding any of these alleged hazards.

Had she contacted either one of us, she would have learned the following (all numbers correspond to the original charges):

HEALTH

1. The lab pumice pan is changed daily by our denture technician, Dionne. Pumice is not "pumus," as the employee who reported us to OSHA had written. To us, her ignorance of the correct spelling implied that she may not have had vast dental knowledge. We used this as a clue to pinpoint the employee we thought might have turned us in. Interestingly enough, she quit her job with us the week of the inspection.

Also, our lab is biohazard-free. The ladies (Dionne and Mary) don't touch any biohazardous materials. We sterilize everything going into the lab. This goes for both the new and old labs.

2. Our handpieces were sterilized after every procedure by Jenny, our head of sterilizing at that time. Jenny could have told her our correct protocol. (Fig. 3.1.)

3. The doctor who refused to wear gloves began wearing gloves when the BBP standard went into effect. Also, everyone had clinic jackets, but were required to wear them starting only on the effective date, July 6, 1992. Masks and goggles were available for those who did want to wear a face shield. All protective equipment was required of all employees starting July 6, 1992, the date the BBP standard became effective.

4. Even the OSHA inspector was surprised that the complaintant believed our coffee area to be in the sterilization lab. It was not.

SAFETY

1. There was no second exit from the basement. This is true. (This was not a violation of the BBP standard.) How did we fix this? We moved into our new, larger office, in which all rooms are on one level.

Given the date this complaint was filed (one day after the BBP standard became effective) and given the trumped-up charges, it's obvious the employee held a grievance. This is unfortunate, but it happens.

Jerry and Schmidty sat in the doctor's office and hashed out some details. Jerry wanted to inspect the operatory; Schmidty said that would be impossible as it would violate patient privacy. Schmidty wanted to be included in staff interviews; Jerry said that was impossible because Schmidty was the owner of the business.

When they appeared to reach a stalemate, each decided to get advice. Jerry called his supervisor in Des Moines and Schmidty called the ADA's legal department in Chicago. Schmidty spoke with Kathleen Todd, JD, who continued to advise Schmidty and me throughout the OSHA inspection process.

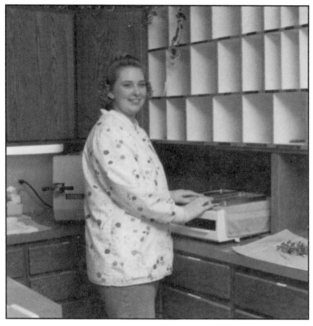

Fig. 3-1   Sterilizing assistant Diana Chudzinski ensures we have plenty of
sterile instruments.

Jerry said the state attorney for OSHA would be contacting us to
explain the laws. We explained that since we had legal counsel, it
would be better if we let the lawyers iron out the details. Jerry agreed,
and we sensed he was as relieved as we were to forestall the inspection.
We guessed that this was Jerry's first dental office inspection.

Kathleen Todd worked closely with Schmidty and me on the
phone, compiling documents and talking about the implications of an
OSHA inspection. She and the ADA were great in helping us contact
OSHA and set up guidelines for the inspection. We had the bonus of
working on one of the first inspections of a larger, privately-owned
dental office so the territory was new to OSHA. It gave us leverage I
don't think you'd get today.

Anyway, when all was confirmed and agreed upon by the attorneys
and Schmidty, the only thing left to do was to wait. And wait, and
wait...

The Inspection

Jerry came back weeks later when we least expected him. I had just finished a prophy—I had my Iowa license now—and was walking my patient to the front desk. Out of the corner of my eye I recognized a face but couldn't place it. I dismissed my patient and discreetly stole a glance at the blond, blue-eyed gentleman in the reception room.

Then it hit me like a lightening bolt. Jerry's back. And he brought his boss with him!

Over the time leading up to this event, we had hammered out the details of the inspection. Jerry would be allowed to observe the operatories if he dressed in a clinic jacket to appear as if he were a visiting dentist. This would ensure that patients would not be alarmed by his presence and he could move throughout the area incognito.

Also, among the ADA, OSHA and our office, it was decided that I could act as employee representative (through a staff election) and be present during staff interviews. This would, of course, be at the discretion of the staff member being interviewed.

As a dental hygienist and employee of a dental office you have certain rights during an OSHA inspection. Number one, if you want to speak with an inspector privately and alone, you may do so. Simply approach the inspector and tell him you'd like to be interviewed. Most likely, he will approach you anyway. Do not be intimidated simply because he or she is a government official. You do not have to feel pressured to help them in any manner. The only person whose best interest is served by assisting the inspector is the owner of the practice. You are under no obligation to kowtow to the inspector's demands.

These are your rights when an OSHA official asks to interview you:

1. Refuse to be interviewed. Refuse to answer any questions. You have the right to be silent. You don't have to help or hinder the inspection with interjections of your own. Just go about your daily routine and remember your BBP standard protocol.

2. Have an employee (or union) representative with you during an interview. This is particularly helpful if that person understands technical government language. Sometimes inspectors use jargon

only governmental workers understand. It might be confusing and cause misinterpretation of facts.

3. Request a private interview with the inspector. You may ask questions to the inspector or ask for clarification of your rights.

At no time during an interview with an OSHA inspector will your employer be present. You are protected at all times from retribution for anything you say during an interview or an inspection. Your employer may not penalize you in any way for honest disclosure of office policy.

During our office inspection Jerry asked 15 staff members (half of our office) for interviews. Three declined. Six preferred to interview in private and six desired my presence during the interview.

I am bound by a great sense of moral integrity, as well as by law, never to reveal what was said in those six interviews—most especially not to Schmidty. I will say, however, that my role during the interviews was as both supporter and interpreter. OSHA inspectors can get a little intense and technical.

It also helps to have a sense of humor.

Jerry was in the basement lab speaking with the guys and gals down there. I stood behind him waiting to escort him upstairs. He reached into his pocket and pulled out a mint and popped it into his mouth.

"Jerry," I whispered, "we don't allow eating in the labs."

He smiled. Did he blush?

To this day, I can't decide if he did that on purpose.

Four Months Later...

I ran into Schmidty's office, "Dad! Guess what? Jerry just called! We didn't have a single violation of the BBP standard!"

It was a victory for the entire office. We earned it. Months of hard work went into planning and plotting, arguing and sweating over how to implement that BBP standard. And we did it.

According to an article by Kathleen Todd in the *Journal of the American Dental Association* (JADA) published in January 1993, we were the first dental office in the country to pass an OSHA inspection without a single violation of the BBP standard.

It is possible to work in a completely OSHA-approved office. It just takes teamwork. Put in your two cents. Offer ideas. Give your time and talents to ensure your work environment is safe. After all, you are the one who benefits by having a safe, OSHA-approved office.

Exposure Control Plan

Do you wonder if your employer is following the BBP standard to the letter? Have you read it?

Dental hygienists would be well-served to understand the BBP standard. Since it's written in government verbiage and not everyone has the time to decipher, we'll stick with the main points of the standard, in clear, plain English.

Highlights of the BBP Standard

IMPORTANT DEFINITIONS

BOPIM: Blood or other potentially infectious materials like body fluids, body products, and body parts.

Exposure Control: Infection control.

Exposure Incident: Contact with BOPIM through eyes, mouth, other mucous membranes, broken skin, or parenterally.

Engineering Controls: Items such as Sharps containers that remove likelihood of an exposure incident in the workplace.

PPE: Personal protective equipment such as gloves, masks, and eyewear (or face shield), clinic jackets.

Regulated Waste: BOPIM and items (2 x 2s, cotton rolls, *et al*) that contain BOPIM and when squeezed would release BOPIM. Rule of thumb: if it is saturated with BOPIM, it is regulated waste or biohazardous waste.

Universal Precautions (UP): Treating all patients as if infected with hepatitis B virus (HBV) or HIV.

Work practice controls: Item such as needle cappers that reduce likelihood of exposure incidents in the workplace.

The Exposure Control Plan

The Exposure Control Plan (ECP) is a written plan stating the manner in which the office is adhering to the BBP standard. It will include three classifications of employees at risk for exposure: all, some, or none. In other words, dental hygienists would fall under the category of "all employees are potentially exposed."

The ECP should also contain a list of exposure tasks and procedures for the "all" and "some" groups. This is a list of job duties in which exposure may be likely. An example would be the task of chairside instrumentation.

Another item needed in an ECP is a notation on how the BBP standard will be implemented—the employer states how she's going to protect you by following the rules. It can include a listing of every possible protection device and its location in the office, as well as step-by-step guidelines of how to perform each duty.

A mapped-out plan for each employee to follow during an exposure incident should appear here as well. In our office, our keyword is BLAB: make the wound BLeed, Apply alcohol or bleach, Blab to your co-worker to get coverage for your position, and blab to the front desk to give you a red card and call the hospital.

We have an agreement with a local hospital that when an employee experiences an exposure incident, he or she gets immediate attention from the emergency room. A receptionist from our office calls to notify the hospital that an employee has been exposed and is coming right over. The receptionist secures transportation for the employee and hands her a red card.

The red card (the size of a business card) gives her priority in the emergency room and alerts staff there to the incident. The hospital then takes care of the HBV antibody (anti-HBs) titer, HIV testing, and HIV counseling that is required by law. Employees feel comfortable because they have a plan of action should the unthinkable happen.

The ECP is available to read at any time. You should read your office's ECP at least once. It's your right. Also, it's usually updated yearly or as the need arises, so you might want to peruse it once a year to ensure you have the most current information.

Methods of Compliance

Universal precautions will be used with every patient, every time, no exceptions. Enough said.

Engineering and work practice controls should be in place. This includes making sure the Sharps containers are available and replaced as needed; adequate hand-washing facilities are provided; needle cappers are present; and contaminated instruments and equipment are disinfected or sterilized.

There also are rules we must follow in the work area. We know we shouldn't chew gum, or eat or drink by the chair. We also know that putting on lipstick or balm, or any other cosmetics is forbidden. Even brushing our teeth can get us into trouble.

The BBP standard also states that it's illegal to smoke in the operatory. No lying, it really says this. I shared this joke with a couple hygienist friends of mine and a nurse. We invented the world's sloppiest hygienist. Her chair is a pig sty, with bloody 2 x 2s littering the floor and rusted instruments in her tray. She's a disheveled mess, with a clinic jacket wide open revealing a bright puce tube top, and she has a cigarette butt hanging out of her mouth. Her name is Tiny the Hygienist, and she's the polar opposite of everything that dictates a true hygienist. Not a pretty sight.

Personal Protective Equipment (PPE)

PPE, including hypoallergenic forms, should be accessible in all sizes. It doesn't state that we can dictate color, however. Too bad; I'm really partial to green gloves and a pink mask. Must be a leftover instinct from my preppy days.

Clinic jackets or scrubs must be worn only in work areas, not in the staff lounge, the restroom, or out of the building. Have you ever seen a doctor's office staff wearing their scrubs out to lunch? I have. They all ate pizza. Yuck. Thank goodness we in dentistry know better.

Clinic jackets or scrubs should be removed when using the restroom because the clothing is considered biohazardous. That's why we must leave the jackets or scrubs at work for laundering when we leave for the day. Once worn chairside, they can't leave the building.

Housekeeping

Housekeeping procedures are simply methods by which everything is sanitized. There must be a written schedule for how and when items will be cleaned and disinfected. When we've dismissed our patient, we sterilize the instruments and disinfect our chair. If something gets contaminated, we clean it. Pretty logical stuff.

It also states that regulated waste should be thrown away in an appropriate manner. Regulated waste would refer to bloody 2 x 2s that are saturated (blood can be squeezed from it). Regulated waste must be placed in a closeable, biohazardous-labeled or color-coded (red) receptacle, and protected from spills and leaks. It must be disposed of in accordance with state laws. OSHA has no jurisdiction over disposal methods.

Nonregulated items, like saliva- and blood-coated items, are thrown out in normal trash. Generally, there are few (if any) items produced during dental hygiene procedures that would fall under the regulated waste category. Regulated waste would refer to blood-soaked items used during surgical procedures, as well as any teeth, bone, or other body tissues.

Hepatitis B Vaccination

Your employer must provide the HBV vaccine to you. If an employee declines the vaccine, she must sign a statement of knowledge. It says she understands that through job exposure to BOPIM she's at risk of acquiring HBV. It also states she's been given the opportunity to be vaccinated free of charge but declined. Populations declining the vaccine could include a pregnant or nursing employee, or one who has presented allergic reactions to an initial dose in the past.

It also states the employee understands that she's at a continued risk of acquiring the HBV, which OSHA calls a "serious disease." Of course it's serious, it can be deadly. If she continues to have occupational exposure to BOPIM, and desires to be vaccinated in the future, she may receive the vaccination series anytime at the employer's expense.

Symptoms of HBV. One-third of infected individuals present no symptoms. One-third have mild flu-like symptoms, and one-third have severe symptoms such as jaundice, dark urine, fatigue, nausea, and anorexia.

Training

Your employer must provide training on OSHA and BBP standards as well as an overview of the hazardous chemicals used in the office. You must be paid for this training and it must be offered annually.

If you are being inadequately trained, speak to your employer. Training is an area where hygienists can expand their job classification. We can offer our intelligence and communication skills to better our work environment.

Maybe we could offer to lead office OSHA training. It's as simple as reading the BBP standard and the ECP, breaking them down into easy-to-understand pieces, and presenting them to co-workers over muffins and orange juice.

Dental hygienists are the perfect choice to be the office coordinators for OSHA. We have abilities uniquely suited to this position, such as schooling in science and inherent people skills. We should take to it like fish to water.

If this interests you, speak to your employer about becoming the office coordinator. You'll need to work out the specifics of compensation. Don't set your hopes too high for payment, though additional compensation should be a prerequisite to taking on the added responsibilities and effort. The experience itself can be very rewarding (see Chapter 8).

Latex Hex

Her lips bulged like the Bubba Shrimp character in "Forest Gump." A bright, red rash covered her chin and cheeks and slight welts rose also. Crocodile tears popped out of her brown eyes and streamed down her reactive face. Hunched over in the dental chair, Ginger sobbed, "Oh, doctor, what happened to me?"

She had been in the day before for some simple fillings. This the dentist remembered distinctly. No drugs had been prescribed and no nitrous oxide was given. She was given local anesthetic, a kind she had had many times before. It had been a benign, routine appointment. She was dismissed without incident.

The dentist checked her medical history records. It showed she knows of no allergies and doesn't take any medications. Her blood pressure and breathing were normal today. "Ginger, did you take any medications last night, prescription or OTC?"

"OTC?"

"Over-the-counter, like Advil, Tylenol, cold medications or the like."

No, she said, she didn't take any pills or medications. The dentist inquired about her eating habits; had she eaten things she hadn't before? Again, her reply was negative. She couldn't remember any spices or foods that were newly experienced. She hadn't been exposed to any new environment, animals, or aerosols. The dentist's brow furrowed in thought.

She took a mirror and an explorer from the tray to examine Ginger's mouth. Inside, her gum tissue was inflamed as if she had gingivitis but the dentist remembered her pretty pink gums and good oral hygiene from yesterday. The fillings looked shiny new and intact. She had older fillings, both amalgam and resin composite, that were holding up well. The dentist was perplexed.

Then, an article she had read in a dental journal came to mind. "Has anything like this ever happened to you before?" she asked, hoping for the answer she was expecting.

"No."

Wrong answer, but, maybe it was a communication error. Maybe Ginger didn't understand the question as intended. The dentist continued playing Nancy Drew.

"Have you ever experienced a slight redness, or a little puffiness in your lips after dental treatment?"

"Well, yeah, I guess I get a little red after I get my teeth cleaned. But it's never this bad, this horrible!"

"I know, I know." Just what she was looking for. "So, after your cleanings, and after fillings, your lips may get red, you might have a rash there?"

"Yes, but I hardly notice it."

"Exactly. Until this time. Ginger, it looks like you might possibly have an allergy to latex."

"Latex? That's not the stuff in my fillings, is it?"

"No, no." She took off her gloves and showed her. "These are latex, Ginger."

She went on to explain that some people are allergic to latex. It's almost always an allergy that develops over time and exposure. The first thing she needed to do was to immediately visit her medical doctor and get a definitive diagnosis. A simple blood test would determine an allergy. Also, her medical doctor could prescribe the correct cream or pills to ease her immediate suffering.

The next week Ginger called our office to update her medical history records. She said she was now allergic to latex.

Latex allergies rose sharply in the '90s, and continue to rise. This is most likely due to the widespread use of latex in medical and dental settings since 1987. That's the year when the Centers for Disease Control and Prevention (CDC) imposed universal precautions for prevention of HIV exposure.

UP means that healthcare workers must treat every patient as if he is infected by HIV and/or HBV. OSHA mandated UP for dental offices in July, 1992 with the introduction of the BBP standard. At that time it became a federal law to comply with UP.

Donning latex gloves is part of the protection process. Latex allergies among healthcare workers is higher than among the general population. This could be due to prolonged exposure to latex in gloves and in various apparatuses in hospitals and clinics. But what can be done for someone with a latex allergy, especially if she's a dental hygienist and her career demands gloving?

Well, first it's important to understand the two distinct types of latex allergies. The first type is thought to be a reaction to the proteins derived from rubber tree sap present in latex. This type of allergy results in Ginger's symptoms—swelling, welting, and reddening of the skin. It can also produce respiratory problems and a frightful drop in blood pressure. These symptoms could be fatal.

The second type of allergy is to the chemicals added to the gloves in processing. Symptoms appear as dermatitis or inflammation of the skin. If there is no breathing difficulty and no sharp drop in blood pressure, there is no risk of fatal reaction.

What can be done to combat latex allergies? Foremost is to avoid exposure to latex. Vinyl gloves are the alternate choice for both practitioner and patient. If you have a latex allergy, your employer is required by law to supply you with an acceptable glove alternative.

But be careful. Latex can be found in many everyday products such as adhesive tape, rubber bands, mattresses, hand grips on racquets and tools, hot water bottles, tires, rubber gloves, some shoes, balloons, baby bottle nipples, condoms, and many more. So people with latex allergies need to be careful everywhere, not just in the dental office.

Creams and ointments may be prescribed after exposure to latex for those mildly sensitive. Antihistamines and decongestants can also be used to combat some symptoms. Usually, those who experience the severe, life-threatening allergy to latex will carry an epi-pen with them. This is an injection device containing a dose of epinephrine. It can be self-administered if breathing difficulty occurs after exposure. Most dental offices have an injectable dose of epinephrine in the first aid kit.

As with any allergy or medical condition, it is recommended that Medic-Alert bracelets or necklaces be worn to alert and inform medical personnel. Latex allergies should be clearly noted in such a case, especially if fatal results might be expected. Also, ensure that your patients who are allergic to latex have it clearly noted on their chart.

Latex allergy warning signs are any swelling, itching, or redness of the skin after contact with rubber products. Any breathing difficulty after latex exposure, such as contact by blowing up a balloon or a visit to the dental office, is also a warning sign. If you suspect you have a latex allergy, bring it to the attention of your physician. A blood test is required to eliminate other causes and make a correct diagnosis.

Because dental hygienists are exposed to latex much more than the general population, we are more susceptible to a latex allergy. Monitor yourself at work and directly after work for any signs of an allergic reaction.

For more information on latex allergies, read the "ABCs of Latex Allergy" pamphlet. Send a stamped, self-addressed, business-sized envelope to: Department of Allergy, Henry Ford Health System, One Ford Place, Detroit, MI 48202.

Requested: OSHA Inspection

As soon as we moved into our new facilities, we contacted OSHA.

"I'd like an inspection, please," was my request. No, I hadn't gone bonkers. Any business can request an OSHA inspection. It's an employer's right.

We all knew that our old office was OSHA-approved. That's where we had been inspected and that's where we passed with flying colors. But now we found ourselves in a new office, and we had to alter some of our plans to conform specifically to our new surroundings.

There were logistical changes that needed to be met, like placing biohazard bins on carts, creating a new sterilizing lab, and setting up biohazardous and nonbiohazardous areas. We thought we did it properly but weren't 100-percent sure.

So we called OSHA. You might want to suggest this to your employer. If she calls OSHA, they will come and give the office a "mock" inspection. The agreement must be that she will change any potential "hazards." In this case OSHA will not fine her one cent.

If you are serious about working in an OSHA-compliant office and your employer is committed to it, this is a perfect opportunity for you both. Actually, it's great for the whole office because you get the feel of an OSHA inspection without the fear. Everyone's fears are calmed, questions are answered, and trust is restored.

Let's face it, if OSHA comes by another means and levies hefty fines on your employer, she may have to close the practice. That leaves us in a terrible situation, scouring the want ads. Not a good scenario for employer or employee.

Since moving into our new digs, we've had two such OSHA inspections—one for safety and one for health, although in our state they have recently been combined into one inspection. It's comforting for everyone to know that our place of employment is OSHA-compliant.

A New, Improved OSHA

In 1995, three initiatives set forth by the Clinton Administration redefined OSHA. OSHA had long been a thorn in the side of every employer—even employees felt OSHA was out of touch and couldn't be counted on for protection. This marked the beginning of the end of OSHA as it had been previously known.

The three strategies to set OSHA on a new and better course were:

1. A united trinity dedicated to workplace safety—OSHA, employees, and employers—with everyone working together to find solutions to work hazards.

2. Some good, old-fashioned common sense to update old, confusing bureaucratic rules and paperwork.

3. Concentration on the most serious hazards, rather than bookkeeping or the incidentals.

With the advent of these regulatory reform initiatives, a new OSHA was born. The government realized that employers are not inherently evil and actually wish to provide safe workplaces for their employees. With a new OSHA, employees also realized that they were part of the team. The team included OSHA, employees, and employers.

Common sense was adopted as rule of thumb. OSHA was to eliminate confusing language and adopt policies that everyone could understand and follow. They were to work with businesses, not against them, to determine what constitutes safety for employees.

Results were the name of the game, not red tape. Timeliness was esteemed. Bureaucracy was abolished. OSHA would now focus on only the most serious workplace hazards. The new OSHA is more work-friendly.

For more information on OSHA, you can contact its page on the World Wide Web at:

http://www.osha.gov

OSHA's standards and interpretations are available on CD-ROM. For information on ordering, call the United States Government Printing Office at (202) 512-1800, or contact your state OSHA offices.

Chapter Four

The Next Generation:
Hygiene Assistants and Assistance

"Space—the final frontier...These are the voyages of the starship Enterprise.
Its five-year mission: to explore strange new worlds, to seek out new life and
new civilizations, to boldly go where no man has gone before."

—Gene Roddenberry
from the *Star Trek* television series (1966-1969).

The Wave of the Future

Dentistry, like all industry, is in a constant state of change. Change
is not necessarily bad, either, as change can provide us with better, easier, more patient-friendly dental offices. The evolution of the dental
office and how dentistry is provided has been the norm since the first
dentist opened up shop in ancient Egypt, or even since the barbers of
the Old West extracted teeth. A lot has changed over the course of
time—to say the least—and still, changes will continue over the length
of our careers as dental hygienists.

One of the absolutes is that change is inherent. One of our jobs as
dental hygienists is to accept the change, work it positively into our
profession, and continue to provide the best dental hygiene care we

can. The ADHA followed this line of logic in regard to managed care insurance (see Chapter 2). The ADHA has accepted that (for the time being) managed care appears to be here to stay in dentistry, and that it is in dentistry's best interest to adapt. In fact, on their position paper on managed care the ADHA writes, defending its position:

> *"It would serve no purpose to hide our heads in the sand. ADHA's job is to help prepare dental hygienists to deal with the reality of managed care in a positive way that will help patients and dental hygienists alike."*

This is very well put, whether or not we agree with managed care. Dental hygienists cannot play ostriches when it comes to changes in dental delivery. We must accept, adapt, and act according to changes that will affect our profession. Once upon a time sit-down dentistry was considered an oddity. Every practitioner stood at the chair. Not today. Most dentists prefer to recline their patients and practice while sitting on a stool.

Another dentistry-altering change was the advent of the dental assistant. Four-handed, even six-handed dentistry was once a novelty. Now it's commonplace. There have been multitudes of changes in the profession of dentistry including the introduction of dental hygienists at the turn of the twentieth century. Keep in mind that our profession will change, we will change, and in order to keep up with the times an attitude of acceptance and adaptation will be extremely beneficial.

This is not to say that all new ideas are good ideas. We are educated, bright individuals who have the ability to seek knowledge regarding latest trends. We can decide for ourselves whether or not we choose to embrace or shun thoughts, ideas, and expressions that may change our profession. It's in our hands what we accept and what we deny. We must be careful, though, because usually majority rules in such cases and change may be thrust upon us, willing or not. The best course to take is to be open to innovations in dental hygiene and dentistry in general as the latest trend may be the next dental benchmark.

Hygiene Assistants

As hygiene develops as a profession, more of us will have our own assistants. Hygiene assistants can take on many forms, from full-fledged assisting (which constitutes four-handed hygiene) to a chair scrubber and many forms in between. During our hygiene careers most of us will have access to an assistant who does more than disinfect our chair but may not assist us chairside.

In our office, our hygiene assistant, Torey, helps with just about every aspect of hygiene. Her main function is that of a hygiene coordinator. She keeps us on time by helping with a variety of functions including polishing, dismissing when necessary, charting, and computer work. Her hygiene assistant job title is really incomplete. She coordinates our department.

Her number-one objective is to prioritize hygiene activity. She knows each of our schedules and at what point in a prophy we stand, which is no easy task because each hygienist practices a tad bit differently. She coordinates and jumps in as needed, leaving the others to fend for themselves if someone requires more assistance. We understand this and accept the fact we may be solo for a while.

If Patti is running behind and her next patient needs bitewings, Torey will go ahead and take the x-rays and seat the patient in another chair. If Eileen is placing sealants, I may have to disinfect my own chair because Torey will be chairside, assisting the seals. When Barb or Allison need charting, Torey's there to enter their verbal commands of both restorative and perio charts into the computer. One of us can pitch in and perform charting if Torey's assisting a difficult Cavitron patient. As Deb finishes her patient, Torey's got the charges, notes, and Periodontal Screening and Recording (PSR) scores entered into the computer as well as the recall appointment made.

In our office, our hygiene assistant has a protocol list to follow. This is how it reads:

1. Prioritize at all times. Start with the highest priority and work down from there. Then prioritize all over again. This should be an ongoing process.

2. Know the status of each hygienist's schedule. Help to keep them on schedule by dismissing patients, or assisting while the dentist performs exam, or finishing the prophy with coronal polish, flossing, and fluoride treatment.

3. Enter the perio and tooth charts in the computer for each patient.

4. Enter the charges and schedule recall appointments and operatory appointments, if needed, in the computer for each patient.

5. Enter treatment plans in the computer as needed, or enlist the aid of a doctor's assistant to enter the treatment plan.

6. Clean chairs; set up chairs as needed.

7. Check stock status in hygiene and x-ray at the beginning and end of each shift so replenishing is not needed while assisting.

8. Take and develop x-rays as needed to help the flow in x-ray.

9. Early shift: set up chairs; stock shelves; review schedules; prepare for the day (i.e., look for sealants, root planings, and any other appointments that may take special setups or extra help.)

10. Late shift: clean suction with Clean'n'Clear; wipe down chairs; and (after the last patient has left the room) raise chairs. Also check stock and tidiness of the hygiene and x-ray rooms.

11. Keep root planing kits correctly together and bagged separately.

12. If not needed in hygiene room, help out in operatory. Hygiene assistants have the right to say "no" to helping out in the operatory if they are needed in hygiene. Gentle Dental promotes a work atmosphere of team involvement. We help each other as needed.

In a multiple-hygienist office, hygiene assistance can be a saving grace. The assistant also acts as a mediator for interaction among the six hygienists. It is difficult for six strong-willed, independent women to work closely together without some sort of a buffer to aid in communication. A hygiene assistant can explain any misunderstandings and alleviate ruffled feathers.

A hygiene assistant works hard. As practitioners, hygienists naturally demand perfection and insist on the utmost care for their patients.

We keep our assistant running to make the most of every minute our patients are seated in the chair. Without this assistance we would have less time to spend with the patient teaching, informing, and chatting (the things we do best as hygienists).

Even a one- or two-person hygiene department can benefit greatly from an assistant. Actually, the closer the hygienist/assistant ratio, the more time a hygienist has available to spend with her patient, and the less time she spends away from the chair performing preparatory work. An unfortunate aspect of hygiene assistance is that most dentists can't justify the salary of a hygiene assistant. A larger practice naturally would have the ability to hire the extra team player in hygiene, maybe more so than the smaller offices.

All offices can afford hygiene assistants if more patients are seen because of their presence. A 60-minute prophy could be cut down to 50 or 40 minutes with an assistant, allowing additional patients to be seen in a day. This benefits the patients because when more appointment times open up, patients don't have to wait as long to be seen for a cleaning. Less time allotted for appointments also cushions the "no show" factor. Patients who break appointments will keep the hygienist unproductive for shorter periods of time.

Time spent on the actual prophy and conversing with the patient does not change even if the appointment is shortened. What has changed is the elimination of time-consuming functions such as charting alone; reviewing a complete medical history questionnaire; entering procedures and charges on charts or in a computer; retrieving records of perio and restorative charts and radiographs; and operatory cleaning and setup. When an assistant performs these functions, a hygienist can spend the maximum number of minutes with each patient, moving from patient to patient without disruption for "busy" work.

Other duties hygiene assistants can perform include sterilizing instruments and prepping trays. Hygienists should be concentrating on patients, not running an autoclave. On the average, dentists don't run sterilizing machines, make instrument setups, or sort biohazardous waste. Why not? Because dentists are producers and they are beneficial to the practice only when they are at the chair drilling cavities, talking to the patient, laughing with the patient, extracting teeth, and seating crowns. These functions (and many more) executed by the dentist keep the practice in business.

The same should be said of hygienists. Their main contribution to the practice is done chairside with the patient. All else is wasteful misuse of manpower if patients are neglected. (Obviously, if there are no patients to be seen or called, then filing charts is a better activity for hygienists than sipping coffee.) Hygienists should be treated as producers—not as prima donnas or as if they were on pedestals. Keeping them busy with patients should be the number-one priority of an intelligent office. If producers produce, then the success of the practice is guaranteed. As envelope stuffers, hygienists are an expensive lot.

> **Hygienists benefit the practice most by spending time with patients.**

Another task the hygiene assistant can handle is to make phone calls to confirm appointments and contact patients on a recall list. A nice, pleasant phone voice is all that is needed. It's also financially smart from the standpoint of the practice. It makes no sense to pull a hygienist from production time to wallow in phone purgatory if a nonproducer is available. An assistant—who earns less than a hygienist and who does not produce income for the practice—is without question a better choice for daily phone work.

> **For a hygiene department to be profitable, hygienists need to be booked solid all day long.**

The same can be said of filing. Why would any practice ask a producer to file, copy, sort, or perform any other kind of office task as part of her daily chores? The responsible attitude for the good of the practice should be to have the hygienist booked and with patients all day long. The goal should be to see that her appointment schedule is full from start to finish. If a hygiene department is to be profitable, then hygienists need to complete prophys.

Entire Office As Assistant

A receptionist is the ideal staff member to ensure a hygienist's schedule is always full. If a patient calls in to cancel an appointment with the hygienist, the first step a good receptionist should take is to fill that empty time slot. Every office should have a "call list." This is a list of patients who may or may not have appointments but wish to be seen as soon as there is an opening.

Let's say the first 7 p.m. appointment is one month from today. George wants a seven o'clock time slot, but wants it in less than one month. The receptionist gives George the appointment in four weeks and offers to put him on a call list. If there's a 7 p.m. cancellation, he'll receive a call from the office.

For a call list to work, it must be explained to the patient that whoever answers the call first will get the appointment. That's why it's important to obtain both home and work numbers. Sometimes receptionists leave five or six messages on home answering machines for one opening. Whoever gets the message first and accepts the appointment by calling back will get it. If we can reach the patient at work, that's even better, because it saves them returning our call if they want the appointment. All this can be done while the hygienist is in the operatory performing prophys.

The office that insists hygienists perform a multitude of daily office functions by wearing many hats needs to reevaluate the benefit of having a hygienist on board. Hygienists are paid producers, not office personnel who also clean teeth. If assistants can confirm patients and receptionists can fill openings, the hygienist can remain at the chair, where she is of value to the office.

> **Having a hygienist wear many hats,**
> **impedes her treating patients.**

Office grumblings about hygienists not pulling their weight or antiquated mindsets that hygienists should be doing more (like filing charts) to help the practice, are detrimental not only to hygienists but to individual practices. Employers should be educated that hygienists are producers and are truly valuable when producing for them. We need to enlist their help in training staff to assist us the way the dentists are supported. When we are seen as prima donnas, we don't get the help we need to keep producing. It really is in the best interest of the whole practice to keep the dentist and hygienist at the chair with patients and the dentist is the logical choice to spearhead this ideology.

Of course, it is not out of line for an employer to ask an employee to chip in when available. If a 50-minute block of time is created by a broken appointment or no-show, then it is an hourly wage earner's duty to help out as needed for the good of the practice. What goes around comes around and good relations with other office personnel benefit us in the long run as well as expose our character. The character of a person is revealed through actions, not words. We also help out others because when we need the help, we certainly appreciate it. However, the goal is to prevent no-shows in the first place so that down time is never an issue.

Because of the size of the hygiene department in my office, uninformed dental professionals in the community—and beyond—accuse us of running a prophy mill. However, with our setup we are able to spend more time with our patients, interacting and creating those special bonds that keep them returning to us for treatment. We are free to chat with our patients, teach home care, or discuss treatment because there are others to do the work that takes us away from patients (Fig. 4.1).

> **Hygiene assistants allow us to spend more time with our patients.**

Speaking of communication, when conversing with patients while chairside, the removal of a mask is perfectly in line with OSHA regulations as long as we are not actively performing treatment. When a hygienist is not physically working on a patient, there is no chance of contamination. When speaking with a patient in the conference room, we don't wear a mask. The same can be said when you raise a patient in the chair to discuss prescriptions, oral health status, or treatment plans.

When a patient is raised in a chair, no treatment is being performed and the tray is pushed away. They might as well be sitting in the reception room. We are speaking to them normally without risk of infection so dropping the mask is not only acceptable, it's appropriate. There is no worse barrier to proper communication than a dental mask. When we communicate with our patients, we must make sure they hear us and understand us. In order to do that, we must remove our masks so they don't miss a thing. Their health can be at stake.

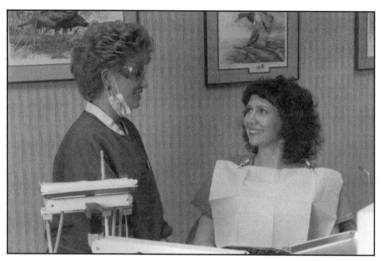

Fig. 4-1 Hygienist Barb Hoppe spends quality time with patient Eileen Tosh.

Dental offices can be complicated places to work. Hygienists daily perform a multitude of tasks not in the least bit related to actual hygiene. This trend will change as hygienists come to be seen as true producers in the office, filling a niche more in line with dentists (producers) than assistants (support personnel). That is why the hygiene department is going to increasingly rely on support from other areas of the dental office, much as the dentist now does. This added assistance will allow us to return to executing hygiene.

The front desk will handle medical histories, payment, insurance claims, appointments, updates, checking in, checking out, and numerous other business functions. The hygiene assistant will take care of entering charting and charges, taking x-rays, disinfecting chairs, putting together instrument setups, keeping hygiene on schedule, acting as liaison between hygiene and the other departments (business, operatory, labs, sterilization), and many other tasks. These assignments allow hygienists to spend more time at the chair, doing what they do best: hygiene.

More personnel, coupled with computers, will ease the difficult work situation of multi-tasked hygienists in a dental office. This situation will also allow more patients to be seen within a work day without compromising patient care in the least. Practitioners will have more time to spend with more patients and all the work will get done. This really benefits a hygienist. Our time is better spent gabbing with Maeve about her trip to Ireland than filing charts in a back room.

Hygiene assistance represents an assistant, or the entire office, helping the hygienist spend more time with her patients.

Progressive dentists have known what mainstream dentists are now learning: the best way to utilize a hygienist is to put her with patients. She's a producer; let her produce. Let her socialize with the patients. Patients know her, they like her, and even if they have no idea which dentist is theirs, they'll keep coming back because of the hygienist.

Patients recognize their hygienists. Hopefully, they spend more time with her than any other person in the dental office (zero decay equals no appointments with the dentist). The hygienist has forged a friendship, a special bond, with these individuals. Patients want to spend time talking with her when they come in. They're disappointed if she's in the other room filing or spending time writing notes. They desire her full attention and with the help of support personnel, such as assistants and business staff, patients will receive it.

Two-Chair Hygiene

One paradigm for hygiene assistants involves an active assistant aiding the hygienist during a prophy. Much as the dentist now employs an assistant, the hygienist could work with an assistant in a two-chair hygiene situation. This is extremely controversial to most hygienists but this type of assisted hygiene is currently performed by some very successful hygienists.

The normal layout is to have the hygienist booked for two chairs with appointment times staggered. Her assistant is hers solely and they both treat each patient. The hygienist concentrates on charting, probing, scaling, interacting with the patient, assisting during the exam,

Hygiene Assistant's Duties	Hygienist's Duties
1. Greet and Seat Patient	1. Restorative Charting
2. Radiographs	2. Probing/PSR
3. Polish and Floss	3. Scaling
4. Home Care Instruction	4. Present for Exam
5. Enter Charges	5. Review Treatment
6. Dismiss Patient	6. Interact with Patient
7. Disinfect Chair	7. Enter Notes

Figure 4.2. Hygiene Assistance: Two Chair Version

and offering home-care recommendations. Her assistant exposes necessary radiographs, seats the patient, enters charting for the hygienist, polishes, flosses, interacts with the patient, performs home care instruction, and dismisses the patient. (Fig. 4.2.) They both would be responsible for completing the prophy by working independently as well as side-by-side.

The controversy lies in how much control hygienists feel comfortable giving to an assistant. The first criterion for this situation to work is that the hygienist must implicitly trust the assistant. There has to be excellent communication between the two and they must forge a trusting professional relationship. Only when the hygienist feels extremely comfortable working with her assistant will this scenario work.

Most hygienists complain that the patient might feel slighted. This is especially true of hygienists who for years have created special bonds with their patients. A practice that employs this method initially runs the risk of alienating loyal patients. When a patient expects to spend time with her hygienist talking about their mutual love of cats, she may feel abandoned when the hygienist leaves for another patient and the assistant comes in to finish the cleaning—it's a natural feeling.

This paradigm may work best if the hygienist is new to the area or new to the practice. She hasn't had time to instill certain expectations into her patients about the appointment routine. Coming in fresh—

and expecting it to work—will aid the success of the program. If the hygienist has an "it will fail" attitude from the start, chances are it will. It's amazing how prophetic our thoughts can be, whether positive or negative. If you think you can, then you can; but if you think you can't, you will fail.

What if the patients complain? Mostly, they are just confused. This is a new way to get their teeth cleaned. It's important to point out the positive aspects. "You're lucky, both my assistant, Ginger, and I will meet your needs today," or, "You're fortunate to have all this attention today." Use whatever wording works best for your professional demeanor. We all have our own unique manner of talking to our patients. The key is to remain positive and point out the good aspects to the patient.

As was stated earlier, this type of hygiene is not for everyone. It takes a certain hygienist mindset to work a two-chair schedule. As with every work situation there are good points and bad points. The benefits to the practice are apparent. There is economic advantage to hiring a hygienist at a certain salary and an assistant at another salary and having them complete double the amount of prophys one hygienist could do alone. It's good for the practice financially. If the hygienist is on any type of bonus program or commission, it's good for her paycheck, too. Even if she doesn't benefit directly from each prophy, by working for a profitable practice she will be able to take advantage of raises and increased benefits.

One important benefit to the patient is that by opening up a second chair, more appointment times are available. Instead of seeing one patient during the patient's lunch hour, the hygienist can now see two. This eliminates needless waiting for appointments. When patients call in for a cleaning, they deserve to be seen within a reasonable amount of time—not three months from now but in the next week or so. If producers are solidly booked months in advance, experts warn, then something is wrong—it usually means more staff is needed. When patients call in, they should be able to obtain an appointment without a long wait. It's courteous as well as good business practice.

There's unrest about two-chaired hygiene, though, as if hygiene assistants take jobs away from dental hygienists. In order to believe that, one has to assume that there is a limited amount of available resources. This is false thinking. It relies on the assumption that there is a limited number of people who seek dental care and, therefore, limited dollars to be spent on dental care. That is not necessarily true.

There is practically an unlimited patient base out there, waiting to be tapped. Fifty percent of the population of the United States currently does not seek routine dental care.[4] This is a vast untapped market that needs to be explored and hygienists are the obvious profession to educate the public about preventive dentistry. There are not currently enough dental resources to handle the influx of patients who will seek preventive dental care services in the new century. Innovative ideas such as a two-chair hygienist will ease some of the strain on dentistry.

Fifty percent of Americans do not seek routine dental care.

The ADHA predicts that between the years 1992 and 2005 the number of new jobs for dental hygienists will increase by 41%. That means there will be 40,000 new openings for dental hygienists into the new century. This incredible growth rate for our profession emphasizes that there are nearly unlimited dental patient resources in the United States.

Four-Handed Hygiene

Even more controversial than two-chaired hygiene is the concept of four-handed hygiene. Four-handed hygiene means four hands and one patient. This is truly hygiene assisting. Perhaps we all perform it from time to time when we have a difficult Cavitron patient needing suction, or when we are placing sealants. The hygienist and her assistant work synchronically. They form a partnership and work together expediently. The assistant's duties encompass charting, suctioning, entering charges and notes, and handing instruments. The hygienist and her assistant are a team working side-by-side (except that the assistant is subordinate to the hygienist).

One plus to this type of hygiene is that the appointment should, in theory, take less time. Less time for the hygienist at the chair, less time for the patient to get teeth cleaned. A 60-minute appointment could perhaps take 40 minutes. This allows the hygienist to schedule more patients in one day so patients who call for appointments can be seen in a timely manner.

The downside to this type of hygiene is that it takes an extremely special duo of hygienist and assistant. Not all independent, strong hygienists can handle such an intense working relationship. One aspect that sets hygienists apart is that they work well independently and four-handed hygiene goes against that. There's not much independence when two are always at the chair.

Another downside is that it could be economically detrimental to the practice. The assistant and hygienist must see at least half again as many patients as the hygienist does alone, just to break even. Unless this is an arrangement the hygienist absolutely must have, it may not be beneficial to the practice.

Yet another detriment to this type of hygiene is that the patient may feel overly dominated by two people at the chair. Patients may feel the two are "ganging up" against them. In fact, home care instruction could turn into an interrogation. While it may work perfectly in law enforcement to have a "good" cop, "bad" cop approach, it's not effective on a daily basis in hygiene. Once in a blue moon a certain hygienist and I will play this good cop, bad cop routine with just the right patient (I emphasize, just the right patient)—to positive results—but routinely, it's not wise.

Four-handed hygiene seems to work best when used in special circumstances such as cleaning the teeth of a severely handicapped individual, a mentally unstable person, one who has a motor physical disorder, a small child who is unruly or needs sealants, or a multitude of other individuals who need extra care and attention. Generally, whether four-handed hygiene works in a normal practice setting is questionable.

Assistance vs. Assistants

Hygienists will come to be seen as true producers in the office. Our practice of hygiene will be seen more on par with dentists, who are producers, than as employees who are merely part of the dental support team. That is why hygienists will rely on support from other areas of the dental office—receptionists, office managers, business staffers, assistants, and hygiene assistants. These employees will offer the assistance we need to perform our jobs.

We should be thinking in terms of hygiene "assistance" rather than the traditional "assistants." Obtaining the necessary assistance to practice hygiene will involve relying on others in the office to help as needed. They will also be called on to assume duties traditionally delegated to hygienists but which constitute nonproductive work—in other words, work that does not realize profit.

This is a call to hygienists to work smarter, not harder. To practice hygiene with the utmost integrity does not mean that every single function relating to the prophy must be performed by the hygienist. It's difficult to imagine a hygienist filing insurance claims or accepting payment. There are many tasks others can handle, including sterilizing instruments, taking a health history, reviewing a treatment plan, or even cleaning toilets. Remember that there are other trained people in the office who are up to these challenges and can execute them perfectly, if given a chance.

Whether or not hygiene assistance includes hygiene assistants is up to each individual practice and practitioner. The point, however, is that by allowing ourselves to be part of the team and relying on others for support, we are promoting the best available care for our patients in a timely and natural manner.

Chapter Five

Patients of the Millennium: Defining and Treating Geriatric Patients

"But he's a human being, and a terrible thing is happening to him. So attention must be paid. He's not to be allowed to fall into his grave like an old dog. Attention, attention must be finally paid to such a person."

—Arthur Miller
from *Death of a Salesman*, act 1.

Meeting Changing Patient Needs

Over the next few decades—maybe over the course of our professional careers—our patient base is going to change slowly yet drastically. Patients will get older, and more patients who previously did not have access will find their way to dental offices. These will include the physically and mentally challenged.

Dental hygienists may find themselves in the position of performing off-site dental hygiene in nursing homes or other care facilities, rural areas of the country, and in impoverished countries. The opportunities abound for inventive hygienists looking for unique venues for dental delivery, but special attention must be given to meet the specific needs of these patients.

According to Virginia Woodward, RDH, executive director for the Kentucky Commission on Women, as we emerge into the twenty-first century in the United States, we will find that:

1. The median age will be 36 years
2. There will be 55 million people over the age of 65
3. The population over 80 years old will total 4.6 million
4. Women will comprise nearly 50 percent of workforce
5. Women will be driving the new economy
6. Women will earn a half or more of the family income (already a reality)

Virginia, during our conversation, said that she sees the future of the world of oral health as a progression toward a "total wellness" of being. In order to achieve this, we need to reach out to those not accessing dental care. This will come in the forms of delivering dental care to homebound and non-ambulatory patients. As Baby Boomers and their parents age, we are seeing the older generations staying at home longer and remaining independent for more of their senior years. Homebound care has exploded in the medical field, Virginia says, and the future trend is to have dentistry follow. Mobile dentistry can be one of those venues.

Virginia also notes that we "need to look at gender issues, (because) we are very gender-related." There should be a flexibility in healthcare, and the issues of particular concern to women and seniors need to be addressed.

These realities call us to look closely at the need to understand the dental needs of a geriatric population that may be confined to facilities or may be physically/mentally challenged. The issues of female patients must also be considered. The profession of dental hygiene is aptly suited to address the dental concerns and needs of such groups.

Beaver Cleaver on Medicare

The aging of the Baby Boom population will affect every industry in the United States. This large group of people—some of them dental hygienists, most of them dental patients—will influence dentistry more than we may realize.

Baby Boomers are the original "Crest Kids." They're the first generation of aging adults to have been widely exposed to preventive dental treatment. They know the benefits of fluoride, because they've experienced it firsthand. They understand the value of dentistry as mass consumers in the dental industry. They will easily go to the dentist every six months for checkups and cleanings.

Baby Boomers have high dental IQs. They are savvy consumers and prefer an active role in determining their dental treatment. They are receptive to alternate methods of treatment and they appreciate the fact that there are usually multiple choices in dental care. Baby Boomers will require continued preventive dental practices as they age.

What does this mean to the dental hygienist? Our regular, recall patients will be getting older. They will expect continued dental prophys and the latest treatments and maintenance protocol. The mothers and fathers of this generation expected to move into dentures in their golden years. Baby Boomers have no such plans.

Treating an Aging Population

As our patient base ages, we need to think in terms of how hygiene needs to change to deal with this population. What special considerations are apparent in treating this aging patient base? There are many, and addressing them all would take a book, so let's stick with the basics.

It's important to recognize the special considerations of an aging mouth. Periodontal assessment and oral cancer screenings are vital. Aged people have aged tissues, which are prone to disease, cancer, and deterioration. Copious notes regarding oral conditions are a necessity. Changes can then be noted and documented. Intra-oral cameras are wonderful tools to document oral conditions, especially when attached to a computer program that shows periodontal and restorative charts and radiographs. Simply by flipping screens, a total oral health picture can be appraised.

The main considerations for treating an aging patient group include increased awareness of oral conditions for geriatric patients;

increased need and adaptation of patient home care; special instructions and special aids; handicap access to dental facilities; and mobile dentistry (at home dental treatment) or outreach programs. (Fig. 5.1.)

Considerations for an Aging Patient Base:

1. Brush up on oral conditions for geriatric patients.
2. Patient home care: instruction and special aids.
3. Handicap access to dental facilities.
4. Nursing home, or at home dental treatment.

Figure 5.1

The regular six-month recall is no longer an adequate guideline for geriatric patients. These patients will perhaps require three or four cleanings a year to maintain good oral health. We'll need to become more conscious of informing our patients of this need, which may be a difficult task. Most people have had "twice-yearly cleanings" engraved into their minds over their entire lives.

> **Twice-yearly cleanings may no longer work; geriatric patients might need more frequent prophys.**

Patients with limited dexterity may need bimonthly or even monthly prophys to keep on track periodontally. This is uncharted territory, so ensure that you and the dentist both use your best professional judgment. Not many patients are geared for monthly visits to the dentist. And if they have limited dexterity, they may also have limited mobility. If accessing the dental office is a major undertaking, maybe other arrangements could be made, such as teaching other family members to care for the patient's teeth, or speaking to a caregiver about the need for oral hygiene.

Other considerations could be your patients' need for partials, rather than full dentures, as they age. Hygienists will need to stress home maintenance of teeth supporting partial dentures. Oral health instruction should continue throughout the patient's life, whether its with the patient or a caregiver. Caregivers should be included in dental conversations regarding treatment and home care instruction whenever possible.

As your patients age they will need to take even better care of their mouths. You can help with your superb home-care instruction. Geriatric patients may develop motor skill problems, which can make home maintenance difficult. Special aids may need to be introduced, and then oral conditions monitored to see if the methods are working.

Also, drug-related oral conditions, such as xerostomia or gingival hyperplasia, must be addressed. Understanding the complexities of drug interactions and drug side-effects could be helpful in hygiene practice. Keeping up-to-date with the latest pharmacological continuing education programs is necessary to treat a geriatric patient base. A complete and thorough medical history listing all medications is required.

Patients in nursing homes rarely receive help with home care. As hygienists, our job is to instruct and inform the community on dental hygiene matters. This includes trips to nursing homes. We can make an enormous difference to nursing home residents' oral health by holding meetings with nursing home staff.

Often, the nursing home staff are so overwhelmed with their daily tasks, they don't have time to think of their patients' teeth. We can teach them the importance of oral care and how it affects the whole body. Holistic medicine refers to overall patient health, including the teeth and gums or dentures. (The word holistic comes from the Greek "holos," meaning whole or complete.)

As the base population ages, the need for handicapped-accessible dental care will be even more apparent. The Americans with Disabilities Act requires the workplace be accessible for employees with disabilities, and most offices are compliant. Also, as physically challenged individuals are becoming increasingly independent, their dental needs must be addressed in a dental office setting rather than a care facility.

The aging population and physically challenged individuals can benefit from a dental office planned with handicap access. Automatic doors, accessible bathrooms, and ramps help both the wheelchair-bound and the geriatric remain independent and functional.

When treating patients in wheelchairs it is important to note that transferring them to a dental chair is necessary. We can treat them appropriately there, without causing undue stress to our bodies or theirs. Practitioners accustomed to working on patients in dental chairs will perform better service when the patient is properly positioned. It allows the hygienist more control and offers more comfort to both the provider and patient.

Another consideration is the amount of time these patients may need. Our appointment times may need to be lengthened to accommodate slower-moving or handicapped patients. Consider tacking on an extra five or 10 minutes for these appointments, or more if home care demonstration is going to include caregivers.

One hygienist in our office regularly sees a lot of elderly patients. She routinely schedules an extra 10 minutes for each appointment. This not only gives her time for logistically seating her patients, but also for the extra chit-chat these patients expect. Sometimes this is their only human contact for the day and they want to make the most of it. They expect the hygienist to have time to discuss their grandchild's latest achievement, show some recent family pictures of a special birthday party, or reminisce about a fragrant flower bed they once lovingly tended. These people need, really need, extra time and they deserve to receive it.

> **A human voice, a touch and a smile is what these people crave. Hygiene is so much more than calculus removal and home care instruction.**

In our town, our office owns the rights to time and temperature. The number is answered something like this: "Good Afternoon. Call Gentle Dental today for quick and smiley cleanings. Gentle Dental time, six-oh-four. Temperature 72." Many area residents call the service to check out the time and temperature expediently. When I found out that some of them were calling the service to hear a human voice, my heart broke. To think that some people are so alone in this world that they'd call a machine to hear a voice is astounding. These are the people who come in with newspaper clippings and a handwritten list of questions. These are the people who deserve our extra time and attention.

Tooth loss is also a consideration, along with periodontal concerns. Generally, the younger the person, the more likely the tooth loss will be associated with decay; and the older the person, the more the tooth loss will be associated with periodontal disease. Educating these patients on the need for replacements, such as bridges and partials, will enable them to keep a working dentition their entire lives.

Hygienists performing prophys outside the office is becoming a mainstay. In nursing homes, on Native American reservations, in rural communities and urban clinics, hygienists are being called to service in nontraditional settings. This trend is growing, with or without an aging patient base.

Nearly half the states have generalized supervision and most others have some variation of that. If dentistry is going to continue to reach out to all American populations, the generalized supervision of dental hygienists is an absolute necessity. If the hygienist is bound to the dentist by a leash and collar, she cannot serve people who do not have access to dental clinics. She cannot offer her services to populations that desire dental care. It's that simple.

The portion of the population that cannot visit a dentist will grow in the next few decades. These people, tied to nursing homes and other care facilities, will desire dental services, and hygienists will be there to support them. We can direct maintenance and recall programs. We can provide screenings and assist patients in seeking dental care. This is not independent practice, this is performing dental cleanings on site under the general supervision of a dentist.

Let's face it, most care facilities are strapped for money. Each one cannot afford to hire a dentist full-time, or even a part-time. With cleanings and screenings, hygienists can fill in the gap, thus providing a bridge between dentist and patient. Hygienists will play an important role in the outpatient dental picture that is developing. This makes the push for every state to adopt general supervision even more imperative.

Hygienists receive financial remuneration at a level which fits with economical service to the indigent in clinics located in rural areas, inner cities, and resident care facilities. These areas, for the most part, cannot afford the services of a dentist on-staff. That is where the benefit of hiring hygienists is realized. One dentist can oversee a larger population, and many hygienists can service each individual area. One or two dentists can make the rounds and take care of dental needs, while hygienists perform maintenance prophys and oral hygiene instruction on an ongoing basis. Working together for the good of these communities and populations, dentists and hygienists can service more people and meet their needs.

> **Hygienists are in the unique position of being available to the community. They are perfectly situated to perform heart-felt service for the public good.**

Our best bet for the future is through ongoing research and study of paradigms that will work. Whatever our patient base, our surest way to best serve our patients is to learn more about them and ways to service them. In understanding our patients we can more clearly see their needs and specific ways to address them.

Women's Unique Oral Needs

The hormonal shifts women face throughout their lives, including the swings faced each month, can significantly affect their oral health. Pregnancy, menopause, and menstruation are all stages of a woman's life where her oral condition can be threatened.

According to Maria McKenzie (an ADHA president and lecturer on women's health), as presented in *Access* magazine[5], very few women understand the need for oral awareness throughout their lifetimes. The vast changes in hormone levels a woman experiences at different periods of her life can drastically affect her oral health as well as her overall health.

As progesterone and estrogen levels increase in the female body, noticeable physical changes occur, including an increased incidence of gingivitis. For teenagers this can be particularly trying. They are attempting to adjust to difficult physical changes that include increased body awareness and overall hygienic concerns, not to mention clothes, make-up and hair considerations. To impress on them the importance of proper home care, which at this age will mean more brushing and diligent flossing, is difficult at best.

When we introduce home care to adolescent women, we speak against a barrage of media and peer-group messages. Those messages can be strong. Ever had a teenager stare at you, glassy-eyed and distant, while you demonstrate flossing? Not a welcoming sight, assuredly.

Problem is, these young women need increased home care at a time when MTV and peer groups are the only ones with access to their brains.

The key to good communication with someone who is aloof, as most teenagers are, is to establish rapport with them. Ask them questions about the things that interest them. One could use the stand-by compliment technique, which works for just about anybody. Who doesn't like to be complimented? "I really like those earrings, where'd you get them?" Another entry into their minds is to ask questions regarding their school, family, or friends. If the harmony develops in general conversation it will facilitate our teaching home care. Only when we've opened up communication channels can we be heard over the 100-odd other channels in their heads.

Pregnant women need increased home care and frequent dental prophys due to rises in hormone levels. It is recommended that a woman receive at least two cleanings during gestation, and some hygienists even recommend four[6] prophys. Changes in the physical health of the patient can greatly affect the gingival health.

During the first trimester, when most women are physically sick to their stomachs, home care can make them more ill. Have you ever wanted to vomit and brush your teeth at the same time? Hardly. We need to impress on them the importance of performing oral hygiene when they feel well. This will require a shift in their thinking, as morning and night, when they've brushed and flossed before, may not be the correct times now. If nausea sets in at 9 p.m. (everyone's on a different schedule; morning sickness does not always happen in the morning), then brushing before bed may not be an option. We may need to open up other possibilities for our first-trimester patients. A mouth rinse or brushing during the day, when they're feeling fit, may help. Anything we can offer to aid in the reduction of bacteria will positively affect their oral conditions.

Second- and third-trimester pregnant women may or may not have the same considerations as first-trimester women. They do share the increased incidence of gingivitis and should be educated on home care and the need to complete any restorative work (with their physician's approval, of course). There have been studies that suggest a connection between periodontal disease and premature, low-birth-weight babies.[7] Babies born presenting these conditions run the risk of health abnormalities, lowered immune systems, and even death, although it is not known how the presence of periodontal disease in the mothers relates to their babies' states of delivery. Periodontal disease itself may not even be the causal factor. But researchers warn that any infection, such as periodontal disease, can place a developing fetus at risk. More research needs to be done in this area.

Gestational gingivitis is the main worry of most expectant mothers. We all see the distressed first-time mothers-to-be, who can't figure out what's happening to their mouths. ("Nothing happened to my mouth with the first three kids.") My oral pathology professor once boasted that he was able to accurately predict pregnancy in three of his patients by noting changes in their oral conditions. Increased awareness, coupled with home-care instructions and an extra prophy, should help most women through pregnancy.

For menopausal women, many changes can occur in the mouth from gingivitis to flaky or peeling gingiva (desquamative gingivitis), to even pale or bleeding gingiva. Most conditions are painless but annoying. For these women, hormone replacement therapy (HRT) can either hurt, help, or not affect these conditions. This can be said with utter certainty because the lack of comprehensive studies regarding HRT and menopause is alarming. There is little out there for us to consider when we search for answers regarding menopause for our patients, as well as ourselves.

One of the better resources about menopause is a book by Susan Love, MD, entitled, *Dr. Susan Love's Hormone Book.* The book covers hormones and menopause from a menopausal, female physician's perspective. Susan says, "We don't know whether hormones make you healthy, or if healthy women take hormones."[8] There are other good books out on the shelves, and it is urged that anyone entering menopause, or knowing of someone who is, read all that's available. Only the can correct choices for each individual (whether or not to take HRT, etc.) be assessed.

Osteoporosis is a risk for the aged. Hygienists are reminded that teeth are held in place by alveolar bone and as bone tissue it is susceptible to deterioration. Convincing our geriatric patients of the necessity of eating a healthful diet containing adequate amounts of calcium can aid in the prevention of bone loss due to osteoporosis. New studies reveal different treatments which may or may not be effective in the prevention or the cure of osteoporosis. The wise decision is to have our patients consult with their physicians regarding treatments and remedies.

As dental hygienists we can educate geriatric and Baby Boomer patients on the best course of action for their oral health, as well as their overall health. These are both populations we will be treating as the next decades arrive. With up-to-the minute input from our dental hygiene journals and other sources of medical and dental information, we can best advise and treat our patients.

The Female-Friendly Office

Most family appointments are made by women. Women seek healthcare more readily than men, and women pursue dental treatment more willingly than men. Dental offices that cater to women will see a retention in their patient base.

Ask this question: In what ways does our office cater to women? Some of the ways my office does so is to present a neat and beautiful interior design. It's aesthetically pleasing to view.

Another way is to have equipment that offers instant feedback so that oral conditions can be shown to the patient. These include periodontal and restorative charting programs, where patients can see their charts on a monitor and then take a color copy home on an 8.5" x 10" page of paper. Future charts can be correlated to previous charts to give the patient an idea of where her oral condition is headed. Decayed areas represented in red would be changed to green areas when amalgams are placed. Pocket depths of 4mm at the initial prophy, if improved by the next appointment, would then show a reading of 3mm.

Another program is Computer Digitized Radiography (CDR), which uses 90-percent less radiation than regular dental x-rays. This appeals to women (and men) who worry about lifetime levels of accumulated radiation on themselves and their children. (Fig. 5.2.)

Other office-related programs that appeal to women include: itemized treatment plans with cost breakdowns for insurance payment and patient portions; specialized children's room decorated in a Looney

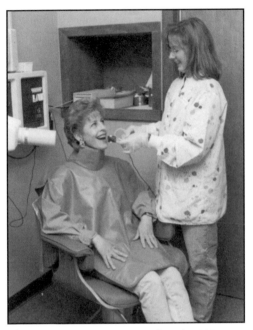

Fig. 5-2 Hygiene assistant Torey Walker takes CDR bitewings on patient Robin Clark.

Tunes cartoon character motif for their kids' dental visits; televisions in the operatories and waiting room; woman-oriented magazines in the reception room; free phone use; vending machines; free toothbrush and toothpaste for everyone in the family (which saves money for a large family); payment options including credit card, ATM, and no-interest payment plans; prizes and stickers for the kids; and early morning and night-time appointments. Obviously, these and more can attract and impress men, too, especially as there are many single fathers out there who look after the dental needs of their children.

Still, promoting your office situation to women will keep your patient base strong.

Chapter Six

The Invisible Uniform: A Refresher Course in Professionalism

"Then you should say what you mean," the March Hare went on.
"I do," Alice hastily replied; "at least—at least
I mean what I say—that's the same thing you know."
"Not the same thing a bit!" said the Hatter.
"Why you might just as well say that 'I see what I eat'
is the same thing as 'I eat what I see'!"

—Lewis Carroll
from *Alice's Adventures in Wonderland*

Friendly Reminders

Time for a refresher course in professionalism. Yes, yes, I know most of us don't need it, but brushing up on our mannerisms and language in the office is not only a good idea, it is a necessary undertaking within the scope of practicing dental hygiene. Practice makes perfect, and in order to be the best we can be, we must constantly scrutinize ourselves as we work. We can't maintain, or even improve, if we're not willing to see ourselves as really are.

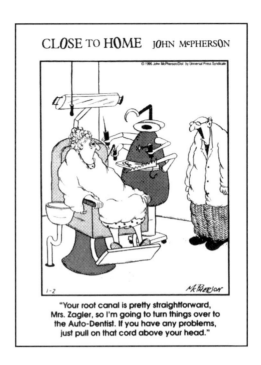

CLOSE TO HOME   JOHN McPHERSON

"Your root canal is pretty straightforward, Mrs. Zagler, so I'm going to turn things over to the Auto-Dentist. If you have any problems, just pull on that cord above your head."

The most important thing to remember is that we are all human: patients, co-workers, bosses, and hygienists. Obviously, as Homo sapiens we cannot claim exemption from the foibles of being human. We make mistakes, we make errors in judgment, we get sloppy or lazy or we just plain goof up. Stuff happens.

Yet, there are steps we can take to not only minimize the number of times we make errors, but also minimize the impact of our transgressions. These steps involve constant and consistent self-evaluation and ensuing corrective adjustment when deviations appear. In other words, pay more attention to the woman in the mirror.

No, we do not want to hear someone tell us how we should speak, what we should say, or how we should act. That's not what refresher courses in professionalism are about. They are about pointed reminders on appropriate professional behavior. When we see the ideal in simplistic terms, we can better grasp the concepts behind what makes a true professional.

Dental hygiene schools teach professionalism not as a course, but as part of nearly every clinical aspect. For instance, we were taught to never have long hair hanging down over the patient. Besides being unsanitary, it's also extremely unprofessional. Everything we learned in clinical studies in reference to our appearance and patient interaction taught us about true professionalism. It may have seemed silly at the time to polish our shoes white or we'd get a check, but our instructors were teaching us much more than how to polish shoes. A neat appearance does not a professional make, but lack of it will ensure professionalism is never attained.

The dress, the actions and the talk of a dental hygienist bespeak volumes of that person's level of professionalism. Envision two hygienists sitting side by side with equal ability and knowledge. One wears old, nubbly leggings, swings her leg that's crossed at the knee and the word "like" peppers every sentence. The other wears new leggings, sits up straight with her legs crossed but not swinging (Emily Post says legs should be crossed at the ankle, but there's no point in quibbling over this), and her speech is relatively free of slang. Which hygienist is going to be taken more seriously?

Of course, this is a no-brainer. The second hygienist will be viewed as the better of the two, even though they're identical. This is what is known as judging a book by its cover. We're all books who will be judged by the cover in which we decide to bind ourselves. This is not fair and it's not right, but it's how the real world works. The world is not a fair place. Yes, we don't like it, but we don't have to like it. We just have to learn the rules so we can play the game. And we definitely want to play, because only then can we win, and hygienists are born winners.

Words Mean So Much More

Glancing up from the computer screen that displayed the appointment schedule in a greenish glow, she spoke calmly to the patient. "I can do you at three."

"Oh?" He blushed as he grinned.

The hygienist looked at him quizzically. The assistant standing next to her giggled. "You're going to DO him at three?" she asked, laughing herself out of the operatory.

Now it was the hygienist's turn to blush. She was setting up his six-month recall. She had meant to sound casual, nonchalant. What came out sounded like a prostitute setting up a John.

"I mean, I have an opening at three," she said meekly.

Luckily, her embarrassment was long gone in six months. The lesson, however, remained. Through painful human errors come our greatest instruction. More often than not, experience is our master teacher.

Correct use of language is paramount to our role in the dental office. We are the team leaders in patient communication. Have you ever listened to your colleagues talk? How about yourself? It can be amusing and fun if you make it a game. Put a tape recorder in your pocket for a day and try it for yourself. The results will be most enlightening.

One snowy, cancellation-ridden day at our office, Jenny[9] and I kept track of the inane sayings heard in the operatories. On a paper towel by the coffeemaker, we listed some doozies. "You've gotta get that sucker outta there," referring to a tooth extraction, was my personal favorite. Another, "We don't do that here"—referring to a procedure we do often—irked others in the office.

No one is immune, either. We all lapse into comfortable conversational styles. Sometimes, it can put the patient at ease. Sometimes not. One person made our paper towel list by telling the patient to "just keep breathing, just breathe." It's pretty hard to imagine a patient forgetting something as vital as that.

But what is appropriate conversation in the dental office? The "big-three-taboo-subjects" rule states never to speak about politics, sex or religion in a professional setting (Fig 6.1.). Period. They have been inflammatory subjects for the last two millennia, maybe longer, and they will continue as such. If you're unclear as to which topics should be avoided, check out the debated topics in your local newspaper editorial pages. Usually any issue regarding abortion, Democrats or Republicans, anti-Semitic or racist acts of violence, or unwed teenage mothers is off-limits, especially if your personal view is implied within the context of the conversation. The wise decision is to speak with your patient regarding your patient's needs, their family, their latest vacation or, when all else fails, the weather.

Do's	Don'ts	Maybes
Patient Name	Politics	Weather
Patient Interests	Sex	Current Events*
Patient Oral Health	Religion	Office Events*

* Current events and office events are forbidden if they contain subject matter concerning politics, sex, or religion.

Figure 6.1 The do's, don'ts, and maybes of patient conversations

Two chairside issues stand out as important: our patient's lives and our patient's oral health. People are naturally egocentric. They love to talk about themselves, hear about their health, and listen to their names. Pepper your conversation frequently with your patient's name. It's like music to their ears.

On each patient care form (PCF), in bold, black letters, is written our patient's name. PCF provide all the printed information regarding last prophy, bitewings, insurance information, and medical alerts. For a computerized office, they are like mini-throw away charts (see Chapter 1). Clips on the vertical light arm hold the PCF in place so all who come to the chair can instantly see the patient's name. The dentist, hygiene assistant, and hygienist can easily see that "Mark" is in chair five. Anyone who approaches the chair can refer to this easy reference and use his name.

> **Patients love to hear their own name;**
> **using it liberally will endear you to them.**

Lest you think patients are going to think, "Hey, this is a scam, they're just looking at my name on the sheet," I assure you, they don't. They think of the PCF as a territorial marker. "Hey, that's my name there. This is my chair. That's my information." It's ego-building and comforting for them to see something as familiar as their names. Quite often, I will return to the chair to find patients intently reading their PCF. Sometimes they act like they've been caught with their hands in the cookie jar. I assure them it's perfectly fine to read their information.

After all, everything printed on the PCF is about them. I encourage them to read it and to ask questions.

In addition to hearing their name spoken, they want data unique to them. Have you told your patient with the heart-shaped second molars it's cool? Or how unusual and special is that rotated premolar? By sharing your excitement at oral discoveries, your patient may join in your enthusiasm. If you find yourself talking about the weather for the seventh time in a day, remind yourself of the terrific twos: patient interests and patient mouths. Hygienists can spend all day expounding on home care and oral health.

But what benefit underlies good communication with your patients? Simple. They'll want you, and only you, as their hygienist. They'll be receptive to your oral healthcare instruction. They'll cooperate and they won't miss six-month recall appointments. They could become the patients of your dreams.

Okay, so not everyone is trainable. There are those patients who, for whatever reason, didn't take a shine to us. Some may be so locked up with fear that no dental experience is going to be good. Some may just be negative, nasty people. We accept that, and go on. Our goal is to be the best we can be with each patient.

Grace Under Fire

Penny saw a patient who spoke only broken English. As a refugee from a third-world country sponsored by a local church, he was experiencing a dental office for the first time. As a church member waited in the reception room—office policy prohibited visitors in the operatory—Penny introduced the patient to a dental chair and dental cleaning. In the process of teaching him home care, she tried to discern his present regimen. Feeling she didn't need the assistance of the church sponsor, Penny didn't summon him and instead asked, "Do you clean your teeth?"

He nodded. Knowing his oral health condition was fair, she wondered what he considered to be proper brushing. "Do you brush your teeth like this?" she asked, waving a toothbrush up and down in front of her mouth.

He shook his head and pointed out the window. Outside, it was a beautiful summer day complete with lush green lawns and a bird chirping in a nearby tree. She thought for a moment. "You brush your teeth *there*?" She pointed out the window at the trees. She couldn't quite grasp his meaning. Did he clean his teeth outdoors?

"Yes, there, that," he said, and pointed out the window again.

Bingo. "You c-clean your teeth with tree branches?" Penny asked. He smiled and nodded. "Yes, yes."

Not missing a beat, Penny said, "Timbo, I have something better for you to use. This is a toothbrush." She then proceeded to demonstrate home care. Later, she brought in the dentist to determine the need for root planing followed by periomaintenance appointments, and if a prescription for Periogard/Peridex would be in order. She instructed Timbo that toothbrushes are much more effective at combating "gum sickness" than twigs. It's all in a day's work.

Penny kept her cool, remained positive and truly helped a patient who regards the use of twigs as proper oral care. Much of what dental hygienists do during the day involves detective work. Like Nancy Drew, we set out to solve a mystery on each patient who sits in our chair. Penny investigated Timbo's mouth and found his home care was lacking despite the fact that he reported that he cleans his teeth. Penny researched and found the answer to the disparity between her patient's report and her oral findings. The twig revelation could have rocked her, but it didn't. This is what true professionalism requires: gliding over the bumps in the road, taking it all in stride.

It is said that the character of a person is determined not in actions taken during ideal conditions, but in behavior during the fury of the storm. As professionals, our characters are considered part of our career personas. As a condition of licensure, we agree to uphold not only the highest standards of dental excellence, but also retain a behavioral integrity within our lives outside the office. For instance, we agree to abstain from the use of illegal drugs. Rightly or wrongly, we must abide by the state dental board's decisions regarding the way we live our personal lives. As licensed professionals, we are expected to adhere to stricter mores than the general public. It is the perception of the board, our patients, and our employers that determine if we are to be considered professionals.

How our patients and our dentists choose to regard us depends, for the most part, on us. Our professional demeanor dictates how our patients, our co-workers and our employers interpret us as professionals. Our attitude and behavior will help us or hurt us, depending upon what we choose to present.

A Code Blue is the ultimate test of professional demeanor. These are truly life-threatening events that require a team effort on the part of dentist, assistant and hygienist. Code Blues can be a true test of mettle. If you can handle a Code Blue with calmness and clarity, then you've got it made. Most of us, however, can get rattled at the first signs of trouble. Very few of us will ever encounter a Code Blue in our careers.

In our office we have a verbal coding system that we all understand (Fig 6.2.). This system allows us to communicate quickly and privately. Patients do not understand the spoken code, so they usually ignore it. Every team member in the office knows each code, so we can say "Jennifer, Code Red," instead of, "Hey Jennifer, you're running 10 minutes behind, get a move on!" Code Red can also refer to a patient who needs to be seen quickly, or needs to get in and out as fast as possible. The receptionist will write "Code Red" on the patient's chart. The hygienist will then know that this is a priority patient.

For difficult patients, we don't have to say, "Doctor, the patient in my chair is complaining about her treatment plan. She thinks that every time she comes in we conveniently 'find' more work." We can say, "Doctor, Code Yellow, regarding treatment." Let her tell him what's wrong with her treatment plan. Mostly, the codes are not spoken in front of the patient, but even if a code call is overheard, the patient will usually ignore it. This is due to the fact that people generally don't listen to what they don't understand.

As described, Code Yellows are truly difficult patients and they can present us with challenges. The patient who loudly yells, "You don't know what you're doing, you're poking me!" when you begin probing is a Code Yellow. So is the patient who threatens to sue the dentist, you, and the whole office if he doesn't get what he wants, now. In other words, these are the times when all you want to do is put down your scaler and go home. The best way to handle Code Yellows is to keep your balance and composure. First of all, take a deep breath. This is no time for shallow breathing. Suck oxygen deep into your lungs.

Then, count to 10—just like you'd do with a smart-mouthed kid you don't want to bop upside the head. Relax, and in a calm almost monotone manner, repeat his offending statement verbatim. For instance, "You said, my shirt hides a pretty big chest—is that correct?" It may shock his ears to know what he's said. Often, a person will not truly understand the power of his own statement until he hears it

Code Yellow:	Difficult Patient: continue with prophy, or dismiss patient.
Code Red:	You're Behind Schedule: shake a leg, or ask for assistance
Orange Alert:	Jail/Prison Patient: count your instruments before and after.
Code Blue:	Life Threatening Emergency: summon help, yell, "Code Blue!"

Figure 6.2. A Rainbow of Codes

repeated. For disruptive patients, hearing their own words echoed back to them can stun them into a less-offensive stance and more submissive role. The way your patient/employer/co-worker (this works for everyone, even family members) responds to your restatement will direct your next course of action.

We have three options every time a patient becomes a Code Yellow:

1. Remain calm, talk to the patient, ask him questions. Sometimes just opening up a line of communication solves the issue. Keep your stance, but see if maybe he really thought you'd think his off-color joke would be funny. If the behavior is so offensive that it's an apology you want, then ask for it.
2. Ask the patient if he wants to reschedule his appointment. Say, "Maybe this isn't the best time for a cleaning for you. Let's schedule this for another day." Give him the option to bail out. Maybe he's really upset over putting his mother in a nursing home and spending half a grand on dental work was not on his agenda. He started yelling only because that's what he does at home. For him it's appropriate behavior.
3. Dismiss the patient/call over the dentist. Depending upon your rules of employment, you may want to involve the dentist/employer in your situation. At our office, hygienists have the ability to dismiss patients who are abusive or disruptive, if we've exhausted all other options. Complete documentation is required, and all other team members who witnessed the event must document it, as well. At other offices, only the dentist can dismiss a patient. Sometimes, just calling over the dentist—an authority figure in the eyes of the patient—can quell an explosive situation.

Speak with your employer about what steps you should take if a patient becomes abusive. As I said, in our office, every hygienist has the right to dismiss a patient on the spot if a patient shows aggressive, threatening or unwelcome sexual behavior. We have the complete backing of our dentists and other office personnel, which is important in these situations. Of course, other venues must be sought, such as establishing a dialogue to determine the problem and offering to reschedule the appointment.

The trick to dealing effectively with Code Yellows is realizing the difference between a threatening patient and one who just complains. A frightened patient may exhibit the same signs and symptoms of an angry patient. Check out your gut instinct. Is your heart telling you he's a difficult patient, a scared person, or a menace? If you can't tell, get a dialogue going. Your patient will reveal his true colors in due time. Communication is the key. The more questions you ask, the better your base of knowledge will be. Get your patient to do the talking.

If he's a complainer, get on with your work and get him out the door. Suffering through difficult patients is unfortunately just part of the job. Dental hygienists are people persons. That's why we got into the healthcare industry in the first place—to help and touch others. Sometimes people seem untouchable, cold, angry, or unfeeling. We can't let these anomalies get us down. We are trained to provide the highest standards of dental hygiene care to everyone, regardless of personality. If the Code Yellow is disruptive enough to prevent delivery of service, then the appointment should end. If not, then we just have to make it through the appointment and hope the patient will be in a better mood the next time.

Scenario #1. Iva sat up in the chair with her knees bent to her chest and her heels planted firmly in the vinyl of the chair. The hygienist patiently explained the doctor's treatment plan consisted of one immediate crown and another "down the road." Iva narrowed her eyes and spat, "Oh, so this is how you intend to pay for your new office. First, my daughter, who has never had a cavity in her life, needs two new crowns, and now so do I." Iva crossed her arms and gave the hygienist a nasty smile.

What would you do?

First, let me tell you what I did, and then let me tell you what would be a better solution to the situation. At the onset of the strife, I defended our office, with gusto. I sternly told her that our office was beyond reproach, that we upheld the highest ethical standards and our doctors were, well, saints. I continued on about how wonderful we were and how every treatment plan was purely upright and honest. This, unfortunately, is not the correct way to handle a complaining patient. In taking an opposing view to the patient's, a hygienist can set herself up for a full-scale war. The patient will become more adamant that her beliefs are founded. This "butting heads" kind of arguing is rarely fruitful. And in arguing inflexibly, the stoical hygienist may appear to be defending the dentist at any cost, regardless of the validity of the contention. In other words, through protesting too much, the hygienist creates the assumption that she really believes the opposite.

"The lady doth protest too much, methinks."
—William Shakespeare, *Hamlet*

When the hygienist defends a doctor's treatment plan, she is defending the office, the doctor's integrity and knowledge, and the profession of dentistry itself. This is an enormous undertaking, even for the most highly-skilled communicator.

A stance of unwavering and domineering defense is overkill, and needless, too. First and foremost, the patient isn't going to listen to a word the hygienist says. The hygienist may just as well orate to a brick wall. Even the most impassioned speaker cannot reach an audience not willing to listen. So, any large-scale argument with Iva is out of the question. (Defending dentistry is important, but as with anything, timing and demeanor are critical; dealing with a disruptive patient is a questionable place to start.)

Here's what would have worked better with Iva. I would have told her, nicely, to take her heels out of my chair and put her legs down. Second, I would have smiled. A warm smile is disarming to an angry person and throws them. They expect their anger to be contagious, which most times it usually is. Instead, they encounter a smiling—or at least a calm—person. Smiling helps us keep our cool, as it's difficult to get upset while smiling.

This sounds absurd and much like a quick fix to a complex problem, but smiling is an accepted countering device. Using it strategically within the context of a confrontation can aid one's stance. Notice lawyers in courtrooms, or politicians in a press conference—they are unruffled and in control. They may even smile, just a bit, to let us know that they really don't take the reporters' questions seriously, or that their client can't possibly be guilty just because Jane Doe saw him pull the trigger. These are trained professionals in the art of debate and confrontation. They remain calm, cool, and collected in the face of adversity.

Next, with Iva, it would have been best to open up the lines of communication. "Iva, what troubles you most about your treatment plan?" Then, I would have listened.

Iva has a beef with the office, and it's important to her that her views are heard. People just want to be heard. As long as Iva didn't upset other patients, or become abusive or loud, it would have been fine to allow her to let off some steam. She was a pressure cooker just waiting to burst. Oftentimes, just permitting a disruptive patient to vent her frustrations will be enough to diffuse the situation.

If she continued to scorn her daughter's treatment plan, I could have gotten the records and found Iva's argument held no merit. Maybe her daughter had numerous fillings in the past few years and Iva was lying. (A word of caution here. When we catch our patients in a lie, we must act with decorum. It is vital that we state the truth plainly, but we also need to be courteous. Every human instinct tells us to be self-righteous and say "nyah, nyah, nyah, nyah, nyah." But when we work, we're not just humans, we're professionals and professionals act with discretion.)

In letting Iva take center stage and expound on her belief of the inaccuracy of the treatment plan, I would have been able to let her release her frustration and calm down. She might have been just fine after that. Or she may have gotten worse, which is the time to end the discussion. If Iva insisted on berating the office and was taking up valuable time, it would not have been remiss to ask her to quit. As dental professionals, we can always use our stock phrase for those who yell, scream, and cause a commotion: "We don't act like that here." (It works for kids and adults.) Then they can make the choice: do they want to calm down and speak with civility, or do they want to vacate the premises? They can either play by our rules, or we can ask them to leave.

(Author's note: Iva and her family are still patients, and to this day, receive treatment plans from our now not-so-new office. While this is somewhat rare, it is also important to remember that every confrontation is not the end of the line with patients. Not all problem patients will leave the practice. Not all difficult people are always difficult. Sometimes, they're just having a bad day).

Scenario #2. Everyone in the office knew Raymond was due for a cleaning that day. The assistants warned Laurie about his erratic behavior. He was a handful, they assured. She seated Raymond in the x-ray room chair and prepared the sensor for bitewings. Her hand was a good three inches in front of Raymond's mouth when he leaned forward and bit down hard on her fingers, and then laughed. If Raymond were eight years old, this might seem like childish behavior, but Raymond was not eight. Raymond was in his middle thirties, employed as a factory worker at a local plant, and had no history (that the office knew of) of mental disorders.

What would you do?

Laurie told him to leave on the spot. She threw her gloves away, whisked off the lead apron covering Raymond, and escorted him to the door. Laurie's actions were the result of a gut instinct. "When he bit me, it scared me. I knew he was way out of line. I just didn't know I'd react so dramatically." She was amazed at her quick thinking, but Laurie was listening to her heart and not her head. Her head might've told her to wait, to calm down. Her heart told her she'd been attacked, brutally. Laurie needed five stitches in her hand and needed to undergo HIV testing. As dental hygienists, we understand the value of our hands, and also the pain colleagues endure when submitting to HIV testing for exposure incidents.

Laurie explains, "Sam (the dentist) and I had talked about what to do if a patient becomes violent or sexual. So, I knew Sam was behind me a hundred percent." This is an important assurance for hygienists, as most of us are women. It's easy to feel threatened with aggressive male patients. To know that our dentist backs us is imperative, even if our employer is female. This backing is reassuring and comforting in a distressing situation. To know that our employer generally supports us over the patient is essential to a healthy working environment.

What if the patient abuses us, then tells the dentist that it was our doing? What would your dentist do? Hopefully, if you are in the right, he will fully support you. If you question this, open a dialogue with your employer. You could offer a few scenarios and test the reaction. If he or she waivers oddly on this issue—such as supporting a patient who sexually harassed a hygienist—it would be wise to question the feasibility of working for someone who would rather pin blame on a loyal, hard-working employee than offend one patient.

There are times, of course, when the dentist must consider both sides of the coin, especially if he's known the patient longer than the hygienist, or if the situation is such that the patient's view has merit. The dentist is also a businessman who must at look at the customer's point of view to see if a compromise can be reached. The patient pays the bills, not the dentist, so not every case is going to favor a hygienist's position. And, as we all know, there are good and bad people in every line of work, which means that there are also good and bad hygienists, whether we choose to admit it or not.

Inevitably, regardless of the action you take with a Code Yellow patient, you may second-guess yourself, and that's okay too. There's not a correct predetermined manner of behavior during a Code Yellow. Each situation is unique and dependent upon our own abilities and attitudes as well as the personality and mood of the patient. The best advice is to act with calmness and integrity, and to trust in your fellow co-workers, employer, and careful planning to help.

Preparedness for a Code Yellow comes through planning ahead mentally by creating plans of action for imaginary episodes. Figure out what you'll do if your patient makes verbal sexual advances, unwelcome physical contact, uses abusive language, or physically hurts you in a deliberate manner. Imprint these images in your mind, then see yourself relaxed and handling them with ease. When the time comes that you need to use it, the mental imagery will be there to guide you through the battle. As with a fire drill, when the smoke starts billowing, you'll already know what to do.

Important note: Ensure your plan of action is supported by your employer. Ideally, you should both have an understanding of what actions are acceptable under certain circumstances. Ask your employer for a meeting to discuss certain scenarios. Have them written down on paper and go over each one, asking if your employer can add to the list. Planning ahead will help you avoid misunderstandings with your employer down the road. You don't want to find yourself on the receiving end of a reprimand for an action you felt justified in taking.

Scenario #3. It's Mike's first visit to the dental office in 15 years. He's 37, in drug rehab, and on Title XIX, which is welfare or Medicaid. He presents with generalized moderate calculus (supra and sub), probe readings ranging from 1-5 mm, and Class I mobility on the lower anteriors. His benefits run out in three days and he has no money to pay for continued dental treatment.

What would you do?

Trudy took off her gloves, washed her hands and buzzed for doctor. She had taken bitewings today, and under the terms of Title XIX she couldn't take a pan (panoramic x-ray) the same day, but she knew it didn't matter. They could not submit to Title XIX for root planing, as there just wasn't time. She agonized over this, as hygienists will do.

"He really needed root planing, but there was no way. I knew Title XIX would pay for scales, so I figured that would at least be a start," she says. "I wanted to do more, but he was in a halfway house. He told me he couldn't afford anything after his welfare ran out."

Doctor rushed in, fresh from the chair. She grabbed his arm, and quickly explained the situation to him in half-English, half-dentalese (that funky language we speak—the one we don't even know exists, yet outsiders can't understand). She told him that root planing was out of the question. Also, with three days left, they'd have to scramble to get him in for any treatment. She thought she could do a scale and a regular prophy, or maybe two scales, depending upon the result of the first scale. She said she'd give him a treatment plan for root planing, should he decide to invest money in his oral health himself. Also she'd offer complete home-care instruction.

"Mark, this is Dr. Petersen, he's going to check your teeth."

The doctor performed a complete exam and supported Trudy's plan of action. He also recommended a couple of fillings and a crown "down the road" on #30. All treatments were presented to the patient, including the information regarding his periodontal health.

Trudy removed a lot of old calculus from Mark's mouth that day. Carefully, she explained periodontal disease and its effects on the mouth, and reviewed home care. Then she juggled her schedule and appointed him for a second cleaning and a visit with the doctor for the fillings. These appointments Title XIX would not cover. She ushered him out the door with a toothbrush and his appointment cards in hand. He came back for the fillings, but not for the second cleaning or crown prep. They never saw him again.

Trudy did not perform what would be described as the most proper dental hygiene care, but she did what she could with what the situation presented. This is not terrible. The patient and hygienist and dentist all worked together in this scenario to provide some type of dental treatment for Mark, even if it wasn't ideal. This is a key point here, because sometimes the best course of treatment won't be the only course of treatment. Learning to alter treatment for the sake of the patient's situation is difficult yet important in dentistry. The most pristine treatment is not always feasible for each patient, so it's not a matter of compromising hygiene integrity, but providing some sort of emergency service to the patient. A full mouth scale will never replace root planing, we all know that. But a full mouth scale is better for Mark than no dental hygiene treatment at all. At the very least, he'll become reacquainted with a dental office. At the most, there could be some positive gingival reaction.

These are scenarios we face every day, as we decipher insurance benefits, determine patient needs versus patient desires, and create the most feasible treatment plan for each patient. Sometimes we do the best we can do, and we have to pat ourselves on the back knowing we did all we could. It's not easy when perfection is the rule in a profession such as dental hygiene. But it is imperative to know that some type of treatment, such as a full-mouth scale, is better than none at all. Especially when you know that the chances are slim that the patient will return for extensive treatment such as root planing.

Thank You

Yes, not everyone needs to be reminded to say "thank you," but if everyone were using the words, then reminders wouldn't be necessary. It's odd that a simple little phrase like "thank you" could be so important, but it is. We need to remember to use it repeatedly with co-workers, employers, patients, the dry cleaner, the postal carrier, a neighbor, and with everybody.

Everyone likes their deeds to be acknowledged. To be the recipient of gratitude is to be placed in esteem. A "thank you" can easily and quickly tell someone that they are noticed and appreciated. It can also ensure these good deeds continue. A person is much more likely to repeat a process that has elicited commendation. If an assistant brings our sterilized instruments to our room, we thank her even if doling out instruments is her job.

Saying "thank you" to a co-worker in front of a patient gives you a double bonus. First, "thank you" in front of witnesses, just like praise, has more impact than a private thanks. Second, your patient notices you are generous and kind. Anything we might do to show patients our good nature will benefit us chairside. They'll like us more, listen to us, and believe we are the professionals we claim to be. Pretty great return for a tiny bit of giving.

While working on "thank you," we shouldn't forget "please" and "you're welcome." It sounds elementary, but let's face it, these phrases aren't used as much as they used to be. Our society has gotten brusque, and our vocabulary curt. Graciousness should be the name of the game for the new millennium. More pleasantries and fewer grunts make for a happier environment, whether at work or at home.

Mirror, Mirror on the Wall

A lot of times we gripe because our bosses, who are dentists, don't take us seriously. If we desire to be taken seriously, then we need to act serious. It's really that simple. Liken it to the maxim that if one wants to make a friend, one must first be a friend. A change in professional demeanor to a more serious attitude occurs both inside and out. Professionalism is more than your physical presence, but presentation is a big part of it. It's all in the package: how we look, how we act, and how we talk. This is what separates the cleaning ladies of teeth from dental hygienists.

Take Linda, for instance, a hygienist in Atlanta. She had been complaining that her dentist was not taking her suggestions seriously. She was fed up with her boss disregarding her professional advice and treating her as another assistant. So she decided to change a few things about her attitude at work. She was determined that her employer see her as an important member of the dental team.

"I decided he was going to start treating me like a colleague," she said, explaining that she changed her office image a bit. "I didn't do anything drastic, but, you know," she confided, "some of us are notorious for the hair-do and nail thing." She saved her bright pink pants for weekends and switched to neutral shades of eye shadow and nail polish. "I wanted to look more serious, more professional at work."

But the physical modification was only minor. Her biggest change came with her attitude. "I asked his advice a lot more and we started having real conversations about dentistry. It wasn't, like, where my husband and I ate dinner, or which show he and his wife went to. It was more dental-related. I'd start conversations about amalgam polishing or expanded functions."

Linda said it took weeks, maybe months to see any improvement or change. She just kept at it, she says. She also claimed it was the best move of her career. "It took awhile, but I had to gain his trust as a peer. I guess he just saw me as an employee before. Now we talk dentistry on the same level," she adds.

Linda touches on the main issue hygienists face in their career. Their closest colleagues, dentists, are also their bosses. This makes for a tenuous relationship at best. How can dentists, who see their hygienists as employees, learn to view them as colleagues as well? It's difficult. Hygienists are inherently subordinate to dentists. We rely on them for licensure, regulation, and employment. This reliance places hygienists in a rigid caste system. As hygienists, we are marked as employees, floating somewhere in space between dentist and assistant. Our duties are dictated by the signature on our paychecks (see Chapter 7).

One way we can bridge the gap between ourselves and our employers is to take action to improve our professional demeanor, both in the office and out. In *acting* as their peers, they will *see* us as their peers. If our goal is to be perceived as dental professionals who understand a great deal about dental issues and patient care, we must keep dentists from viewing us as overpaid cleaning ladies. For dental hygienists to take back the power, the pretty-princess image must go.

The best way for all of us to accomplish this is through self-analysis. We should check ourselves out, give ourselves an objective, thorough, once-over. Is our conversational style, or our clothing style, saying what we want it to?

> One of the best ways to be treated like a professional is to act like one, by opening up lines of communication with our colleagues and our patients.

A friend of mine is in her fifties and calls all her patients "honey." "Honey, you just set yourself in that green chair over there and we'll get those teeth cleaned up for you." It works for her quite wonderfully. Now, if I called *my* patients "honey," I'd either get a proposition or a lawsuit. The key to being the best you can be is to let your true self come forth. Find out what makes you special and then enhance it. If you're a bubbly sort, then bubble away with your patients. It's probably why they keep coming back. If you're empathetic, then empathize: cry with them, laugh with them, feel their pain. Take your best qualities and let them shine for you, your patients, and your employer.

The same goes for our appearance. Did we stumble out of bed, pull on some leggings, and rush to work without breakfast or make-up? Or did we take time to get ready, eat something decent (an orange, cereal, protein) instead of something quick (doughnut, pastry, drive-thru)? Did we take time to look good for the day? These factors can affect how we are perceived much more than we realize. As much as we hate to admit it, physical presentation counts. It's not the whole, as there must be substance within, but disregarding the importance of physical presentation is dangerous. A nice presentation is an open invitation to seek what lies inside.

Be wary of being too trendy, though. Maybe black lip liner with pink frost lipstick works for you, maybe it doesn't. Just because it's fashionable, doesn't mean you have to do it. Let's just say, I don't care how great short shorts look on Cindy Crawford, you'll never catch me in them. In fact, I'd be the one in the fashion magazine under the "don'ts" headline with a black box shielding my eyes.

However, it's not all physical. The way we visually present ourselves is important, but it's not the sum total. There's more to it than that. Our behavior is vital to how we're seen. But how do we know how we're interpreted? We can start by playing detective—getting out the magnifying glass and following bloodhounds. The best way to begin your journey into self-awareness is to start with a problem or a notion of what might be wrong (i.e., "I'm not treated like a professional," or, "My employer doesn't listen to my suggestions.")

Take a sheet of paper and divide it into three columns. For instance, if you feel you aren't being taken seriously at work, list specific examples of *how* you're not being taken seriously. In a column next to those, list actions you can take that might resolve them. In the final column, list other possible explanations for why the situation took place, other than people not taking you seriously. If you have a hard time coming up with ideas for the final column, put yourself in the other person's shoes. This is a great exercise to see problems from different perspectives, from other points of view.

For example, Shelly, the hygienist, asked Martha, the assistant, for help during a difficult cleaning and Martha said "no." Shelly was fine with Martha's assessment of the dentist's work load until she glanced up and saw Martha hanging out at the counter talking to the other assistant. Then Shelly began to boil, as she pictured Martha gabbing away while Shelly was working so hard. Later, Shelly put paper to pen and made her three columns. In the first column she wrote that Martha wouldn't help her with a difficult ultrasonic scaling. In the second column, she devised two ways to handle it: 1. Ask for an assistant of her own (she knew this was pie-in-the-sky thinking, but why not think big?); and 2. Clarify with the dentist when she can expect an assistant to help her. In the third column she wrote reasons for Martha's inaction. Maybe Martha was waiting for a patient who didn't come, or maybe she was waiting for an impression material call from the dentist. (Fig.6.3.)

There are two important lessons about this list. First, it gives us concrete actions to solve a situation as we enact one or more of the actions listed in the second column. Second, it opens our eyes to the situation from a different perspective, as we look at another's point of view in the third column. Not every action producing a negative effect on us is the result of someone deliberately hurting us, or someone being lazy. Just because Martha said she couldn't help Shelly with her difficult patient doesn't mean Martha was just going to stand around and twiddle her thumbs. In giving the other individual a reason for their actions, we avoid blame and move toward resolving daily office issues. Shelly can always confront Martha later and ask (nicely) why

Example:	Possible explanation:	Action:
1. Assistant wouldn't help me with difficult ultrasonic cleaning, even though she was doing nothing at the time.	1. Maybe she was waiting for a patient who didn't show and thought she couldn't help me.	1. Ask for my own assistant, or ask for clarification of when I should be able to get assistance from the assistant.
2. DDS did not Rx Peridex to a patient I thought should have it.	2. Maybe DDS didn't fully understand patient's oral condition.	2. Schedule conference with DDS to clarify his criteria for Rx'ing Peridex.
3. Receptionist did not schedule me enough time for a difficult patient.	3. Perhaps she wasn't aware that the patient required more time.	3. Speak to receptionist about developing a code for patients who require more time.

Fig. 6-3

she felt she didn't have time to help with a difficult patient. Getting it down on paper can also release some of the anger and tension inherent in these conflicts. That way, when the time is appropriate to take action, the anger is dissipated and replaced with clear, thoughtful communication.

In resolving these daily conflict issues we can begin to see patterns that better help us understand ourselves. We can see ourselves for who we are, and then make necessary steps toward improvement. Remember, life is journey, not a destination. The day we stop learning is the day we stop living.

It's Not Me, Really!

Let's say we're perfect. We've done the self-analysis and the diagnosis is splendor. We act professionally, look spiffy, and speak that sparkling tongue of television sitcoms. We're model hygienists. Our difficulties do not arise from patients, spouses or children, but from our co-workers. What do you do when your employer, an assistant, or even another hygienist wears you down? These are the times that test our mettle.

Janice used to enjoy lunch in the break room with Dr. Hemp and his assistant, Sarah. It was a time they could all relax and take off their professional personas. Recounting weekend experiences, joking and laughing over baloney sandwiches or Burger King drive-thru was a highlight of her day. Then the dentist hired another assistant. The new assistant, Carin, now joined them for lunch. Janice knew it would take Carin awhile to fit in; after all, it had been just the three of them for years.

"She was one of those people who knew everything about everything," Janice says. "A real know-it-all. It didn't seem to bother Sarah or doctor, but, well, I can't stand people like that." If Janice brought up her love of dog breeding, Carin would give her tips. "Can you believe that? I was raised around dogs, I now breed dogs, and she's giving me pointers on dog training."

She recounts the time her son was home sick from school. Not only did Carin diagnose her son's illness as strep throat, she also gave her the name of the correct antibiotic to use. She told her to insist the physician prescribe that one for him, because another one wouldn't work. Janice was fed up. She knew Carin was a good assistant and was knowledgeable about dentistry. But it was the know-it-all attitude Carin displayed that drove Janice crazy. She wasn't sure what to do.

Janice, like most of us dealing with less-than-desirable co-workers, has three solid options each time a know-it-all gushes forth pearls of wisdom:

1. Ignore the know-it-all and go about your business. Walk away, or act busy even if you aren't. Make lunch plans elsewhere. Try to avoid encounters.
2. Change the conversation. If the know-it-all gets on a roll, spewing forth tedious information about the cellular phone industry, interject with an open-ended question to someone else. "So, Sarah, what did *you* do this weekend?"
3. Stop the know-it-all in her tracks. When she offers advice, step back or hold up the palm of your hand and say: "Thanks for the advice, Carin, but I've got it handled."

The one option available to us in dire circumstances, is to quit. In exiting to work in another office, we leave a known entity for an unknown. There are no guarantees that our next environment will be better. Sometimes a familiar bird in one hand is better than two unfamiliar ones in the bush.

Those of us who have held many jobs in many different venues know that one thing is certain: co-workers who drive us nuts are everywhere. People are the same, whether you're in an office in Boston or Des Plaines. The perfect workplace is often made by us, not necessarily by others.

Actually, by leaving solely for the purpose of avoiding a co-worker, we rob ourselves of a valuable experience. A great lesson can be learned when we discover how to deal with difficult people. Unless we become shut-ins having no contact with the outside world, we will always have to deal with people with whom we don't get along. We shouldn't escape them when we can manage them and learn from them.

But it's my boss, you say—he acts like General Patton. He barks orders and gives inspections. It's impossible to get any work done. With employers, rules apply differently than with co-workers, especially in dental offices or small businesses where the owner is also a colleague and supervisor. Those are distinct roles, and if employers don't understand that, life can be miserable.

Most dentists know little about running a business, let alone managing people. Let's face it, they've spent eight hard years of college studying sciences. That atmosphere is not conducive to business ownership or employee management. Not all dentists are business moguls (see Chapter 7). This means that dealing with dentists can be tricky. They may be fantastic dentists, but lousy employers. Consider Imogene's story.

Imogene spent two months at Dr. Seltick's office and she says that was two months too long.

"He yelled at me one day for using the wrong pen. The...wrong...pen," she says, emphasizing each word. "I was shell-shocked. These are pens he provides us, but that day it was the wrong one."

Imogene said there were other instances where it seemed like he picked on her for no reason; as if each encounter were a power play. But then he'd be nice again for awhile. She says it was like working with a time bomb. Sometimes he'd be sweet as punch, then boom—he'd erupt like a volcano over inane issues.

"I found myself tiptoeing around him, never knowing if he was going to be fun or furious. It was odd."

Imogene says that it wasn't particular situations that got him upset. He'd explode over pens one day and paper the next, she says. It was inconsistent.

"I tried to speak with him about it. You know, tell him how upset he was making me. But he didn't understand. He twisted my words around and made it seem like I was making the whole thing up."

Imogene says she wasn't. To prove her point, she documented each encounter. She took a pad of paper and wrote down each time he verbally assaulted her. The number of times this happened per week astounded her.

"It was too much. I couldn't believe what I was putting up with. That's when I decided to leave."

She says quitting was the only alternative. She knows she did the right thing in trying to work it out in the beginning. To change, someone often only needs to have their eyes opened to their own behavior and how it affects those around them. But first, they have to listen. If we calmly and professionally try to solve our differences and the other party is deaf to our concerns, we have to explore the possibility that they may not care how their actions affect us. This may be hard to accept, but is nonetheless important.

Dr. Seltick tried to accuse Imogene of imagining the events. This is a deaf ear taken a step farther. Not only is he unwilling to talk about the events, he doesn't even think they've happened. This takes some serious sorting out on our parts. Is he just being true to his male nature, communicating differently than women do? Or is he exhibiting abusive, controlling behavior?

Sometimes the only alternative to dealing with horrible employers is to leave. If they're showing unacceptable behavior, then no job is worth the grief. It's unfortunate, but if you've tried to work things out and it still isn't better, then maybe you're meant for another environment. There's always another job, perhaps a better one (see Chapter 8).

Dealing with difficult people is part of the territory. We're triply blessed (or cursed?) as hygienists. We have patient, co-worker and employer personalities to manage. When they say hygienists are people persons, they're not kidding. But the key to good people skills is realizing when someone is a pain in the tush yet tolerable, and when we need to throw in the towel. There's no easy answer. We have to rely on gut instinct.

The Package

Professionalism is an attitude, a uniform we wear for others to see. How we're interpreted by the world depends solely on our presentation. Every minute detail counts: our conversation, body language and demeanor. If we say the word "like" in every sentence, such as, "I was, like, not there," we will, like, be seen in a totally different manner than if we were to say, "I was not there." It's all a matter of interpretation.

For the most part, dental hygienists proudly proclaim their careers. God help whoever puts down hygiene in front of a dental hygienist. That's why our professional poise is so vital. By standing proudly, firmly, graciously, and strongly we paint a superior picture of ourselves to others.

We're not just cleaning ladies. We don't perform prophys by rote. We don't pick teeth for a living. (Well, okay maybe we do pick teeth, but we do so much more than that, too.) We are intelligent, vibrant beings. We are healthcare professionals. We warrant respect.

Every time we take the extra time to do it right, to look sharp, to act top-notch, we showcase dental hygiene as a career to be taken seriously. In our attitude and poise, we present dental hygiene to the world as a profession, not just a job. We are more than just the cleaning ladies. We are dental hygienists.

Chapter Seven

Not Just the Cleaning Lady: Synthesizing Hygiene with Dentistry

"The first day or so we all pointed to our countries.
The third or fourth day we were pointing to our continents.
By the fifth day we were aware of only one Earth."

—Discovery 5 Space Mission

FACT: We rely on dentists for licensure, regulation and employment.

RDH vs. DDS?

Dentists—those guys and gals with the initials DDS or DMD after their names—dictate the rules and practice of our profession. Without them, we cease to exist. They are our career lifeline...aren't they? Do we anticipate that hygiene will continue as a profession without their support? Does self-regulation mean confrontation? What, really, do hygienists want?

Dentistry doesn't understand that most hygienists do not want a full-scale nuclear war. In nuclear war, no one wins. Hygienists need dentists, and they need us. It can be, and should be, a perfect symbiotic relationship. Do dentists really want to perform prophys? Or, have unqualified personnel turned their patients' gingiva into hamburger meat? That doesn't seem to gel. In recent and past ADA surveys of dentists, dental hygienists are recognized as both needed and desired additions to the practice.

There are some hygienists who see their profession as separate and distinct from dentistry, as if hygiene could survive without dentistry. Other hygienists believe that hygienists cannot survive without dentists, and that the need for leaning on dentistry is vital. Everyone has his or her beliefs.

Sarah Turner, RDH, MEd, former ADHA president, says, "Hygiene and dentistry do not have the same goals." This is neither bad nor good, it's just fact. She wishes for hygienists and dentists to drop the parent/child relationship and emphasize the colleague aspect. She feels that since most hygienists are women and a lot of dentists are men, there are naturally going to be communication problems. The aspect of male/female, and employee/employer relationships, will affect the views and attitudes of both professions.

We need to look at the reality of the situation, where both professions are headed, and what will be best for dental hygiene as a profession. This may be different than what each of us envisions for hygiene, but for the good of the profession it is imperative we stand united on common ground. Only then can we meet the challenges of the future head-on, and mold hygiene into the great profession it should be. If we want our profession to prosper, we must be willing to compromise our individual beliefs for the good of the group as a whole.

First, we've got the perfect balance for a great dental office with dentistry and hygiene. It's a give-and-take relationship that works well, if used properly. Some working hygienists may have problems with their employers, but those differences are mostly clashes of personality rather than true disputes relating to one another's stance on profession-related issues. Rarely do hygienists and dentists battle over professional topics while working together. For every hygienist who continues employment in a specific practice—without want of departure— there is one dentist/hygienist relationship that works. The dentist/hygienist relationship can work well and, with careful maintenance and upgrades, it will continue to work better.

Hygiene fees can provide dentists with a good income. Hygienists take periodontal problems out of their hair. We are experienced, licensed healthcare professionals who, through our regular contact with patients, maintain the dentist's patient base. Some patients see the dentist for only a few minutes, twice a year, while spending a couple of hours with us. We are an important link to the patient, and the doctor knows it.

Likewise, the doctor is our employer and our colleague. He/she gives us a good salary, excellent benefits, keeps us licensed, and provides us a wonderful place to work. He/she offers us patients, the tools and utensils we require, and a stable income. We glean from him/her and share with him/her knowledge of all things dental.

Sounds like a match made in heaven, doesn't it? Then why all the fuss? First, let's see where dentists are coming from.

What Dentists Need

Dentists want a comprehensive, perio-related hygiene department that turns a profit. This is not bad. This is just what they need. They have an entire practice to run, and can't be brought down by what they consider to be a hygiene money drain. Profitability of hygiene departments is a hot topic in the dental field.

Robert Ankrom, RDH, BS, practice management consultant for McKenzie Management, says that the magic number is 33 percent. That is, 33 percent of total office production should come from the hygiene department, and 33 percent of hygiene production should be periodontal maintenance. And, hygiene compensation should be no more than 33 percent of hygiene production.

Whether or not you agree with these numbers, take note that this is what dentists believe. They use information such as these figures to evaluate their hygiene department. You may think this is blasphemy, but this is reality for most dentists. These are their beliefs, and we're well advised to educate ourselves on these matters. Next time an issue of *JADA* or *Dental Economics* hits your employer's desk, ask her if you can read it when she's done. It's imperative that we keep up-to-date on the issues governing dentists. If we don't know where dentists stand, how can we effectively communicate with them? Communication on issues, such as profitability of the hygiene department, allows us to have input into the practice-structuring ideas with which dentists grapple. When we build bridges—instead of tearing them down—our viewpoints can be addressed and taken seriously.

Robert Ankrom says the mainstay of all good hygiene departments is periodontal treatment. Every office, he states, needs a well-defined periodontal program. That's where the expertise and abilities of the hygienist can make a difference. The dentist wants an excellent periodontal system, and who is better trained than the dental hygienist? A perfect symbiotic relationship is the dentist and hygienist working together for the good of the patient.

(On a side note, I asked Robert how many other male hygienists are out there. He says the official figure is 800. I gasped. He said a handful is as many as he's found. He knows two of them well, and has heard of a few others. If you are a male hygienist or you know of one, let me know and I'll pass along the information to Robert.)

By involving their hygienists in development of a well-rounded hygiene department, dentists may be shocked at the great results. It is important for both the hygienist and dentist to realize that they're on the same winning team. If hygienists take control and deliver on the production promise, both the dentist and hygienist benefit.

We have to realize that money is not inherently bad, and striving toward financial success is not a sin. "For the love of money is the root of all evil: which while some coveted after, they have erred from the faith, and pierced themselves through with many sorrows," (Tim. 6:10).

Money is not the root of all evil. The *love* of money is the root of all evil.

A profitable hygiene department is not an immoral entity. It's vital to the survival of hygiene as a profession. If hygiene fails as a business, it ceases as a profession. We don't want to hear that, but those are the facts. We live in a country where free enterprise reigns. If hygiene can't make it, then dentistry is going to seek other options. It's as simple as that.

For those hygienists working in independent practice, or those seeking it, remember that profitability will be essential for success. It is staggering when one envisions that patient fees must cover overhead costs that include, but are not limited to, electricity, gas, water, dental equipment, supplies, employee salaries and benefits, employee social security, taxes, legal fees, repair bills, phone service, and office equipment. Those who think that an unprofitable hygiene department is not an issue would be wise to remember that if it were a separate corporation, the hygiene business would be shut down.

Other options for saving money in the hygiene department may include horrendously shocking alternatives embodied in legislation that pushes for hygiene duties to be performed by unlicensed personnel. This is definitely the wrong path for dentistry to take. This puts public health at risk and must be discouraged for the public good. Patients are never served well by having unlicensed personnel performing tasks that should be delegated only to registered dental hygienists.

Abolishing dental hygiene as we know it will not increase the dental office profit margin. The only way to increase the office profit margin is to turn a hygiene department that's a monetary drain into a profitable office division. Hygienists should be interested in seeing their profession as a productive member of the dental team. When dental hygiene works productively for the dental office, everybody wins.

The dentist is well-served by consulting with hygienists during development of a profitable, perio-based hygiene department. We are the natural choice for this task, and we'd do it so well. We know what perio patients need and we can deliver. We can be a productive member of the dental team.

Yes, it would be nice if we could provide our services for free. It would be lovely if we made fluoride available to everyone, or offered root planing to patients who couldn't afford it. But we must remember—no matter how hard it is for us—that dentistry in the United States is a business. When we deposit our paycheck (hey, it's pretty darn good!) in the bank, we should remember who gave it to us. No, not the dentist, though her signature is probably on it. Our patients provide us with a paycheck.

Patient fees pay our salaries, not the dentist!

Every time our patients come in for their recall, agree to fluoride, accept a perio regimen or bitewings—whether they have insurance or not—it is their payment that makes our job possible. It's the way businesses run, and it's not sinister, it's just the marketplace rule. This is called capitalism, and it allows us the freedom to choose to be a dental hygienist and earn a nice living. In the United States, capitalism is the foundation of our economic system.

Hygienists are nurturing, caring individuals. We want only the best for our patients. We want them to have the kind of care we'd give to the person we love most in the world. We want them to have it all. Unfortunately, not everyone can afford to choose the best care. Some may take a four-surface amalgam though they know that a crown is recommended. Not everyone can undergo all treatment suggested. We have to learn to accept that and move forward.

Say I got an estimate from my mechanic that said everything that needs to be done will cost $1,143. Ouch! My first question is: Okay, what's the really important stuff? Let's get that done first, and the other things can wait. I can live with a broken clock in my car. So, the mechanic comes back and says, it won't be the best course of action, but it'll cost $530. Great. Doable.

Some of our patients view dentistry in the same way. They come in wanting the most basic treatment and the lowest cost. Some patients think dentistry is a luxury. For some, it is. Anyway, the patient sits in your chair and wants to spend as little as possible. Hey, that's okay; she's got school clothes to buy, two car payments and a mortgage to make, and bills that would make your head spin. You and I might even be in the same boat.

Our job is to inform, inform, inform. In teaching her the value of regular maintenance and proper dentistry (porcelain crown vs. pre-fab stainless steel), she will be much more accepting of the proposed treatment. If that includes four quads of root planing, then isn't it in our best interest to see that she follows through? Maybe we can offer payment plans her or put the bill on her credit card, if that would help. Our job is to help the patient understand the need for dental treatment.

It is our obligation as dental hygienists to give her the facts, all the facts, including the fee. Yes, it will cost just under $1,000. That's the fee your dentist has established. Your employer bases that fee on her overhead cost—including your salary—and the going rate in the city or town in which she practices. Her fees are fair. If you do not absolutely, positively believe they're fair, why are you working for her?

Fees, money, charge, expense, it's all the same, however we wish to say it. Performing dental hygiene for free is not an option in non-governmentally funded settings. If you feel strongly about needing to give away your services, I urge you to seek other venues for practicing dental hygiene. The dentist-owned (or insurance company-owned) practice would not be a good work environment for you.

Dentists must look at their hygiene department as a business within a business. Hygiene is a little corporation all its own. It won't close down if it's not profitable. The dental practice can keep it going. But it will be a thorn in the side of the dentist if it's a drain on the rest of the office. And, if it's not turning a profit, guess who takes the blame? We do.

The trick is to realize what dentists want, compare it to what hygienists want, and find a way to meld the two. But what do hygienists want, and does it mesh with dentistry?

What Do Hygienists Want?

Now, there's a difficult and complex question. What do we want? Well, here's the beginning of a list I've compiled, see what you can add to it:

- decent wages
- excellent benefits
- expanded functions
- licensure for duties
- good hours
- general supervision
- self-regulation
- educational opportunities

Hygienists may agree or disagree about some issues, but it's impossible to imagine any of us arguing over the need for licensure for hygiene duties. This is first and foremost the backbone of our profession. How quickly would we be out of a job if assistants could be trained in the office to perform hygiene procedures? To keep our profession alive we must support the ADHA in its fight to prevent hygiene functions from becoming assistant duties. The line between dental assistant and dental hygienist must not be blurred. We must stand firm for our profession. But we cannot be lulled into thinking that we're indispensable.

We could all sit back and shrug off the notion that there is a threat to our profession. After all, we still go to work each day, we still receive our paycheck, and we get along with our dentist. She's not politically active in the ADA, so why should we be politically active in the ADHA?

Because her career is not reliant upon another for licensure. Could you imagine what dentistry would be like if physicians regulated dentists? Think about it. That's a sure way to end dentistry as we know it.

This is no way suggesting that dental hygiene as regulated by dentists is the same, or even close to, physicians regulating dentistry. There can be no correlation. But the point here is that we are dependent solely upon dentists for our profession. We are a subdivision of dentistry. Without dentists, our careers are kaput.

We should be active in the ADHA because it is the only body that supports us as a profession. The ADHA looks out for our needs and acts as watchdog for hazards to our livelihood. No one else will. Do we want to continue going to work, receiving our nice paycheck, and enjoying the benefits of a career we can be proud of? Then we need to endorse the ADHA in its efforts to keep our profession alive.

How could we live with the fact that assistants would be able to perform most, if not all, of our functions? It's unlikely that we could. First of all, dental hygienists would become extinct. Our species wouldn't exist. We would have no voice to speak out. Second, the public health would be at great danger.

If people were aware that unlicensed personnel were manipulating sharp instruments in their mouths, I think there would be a public outcry. As dental hygienists we have had extensive training to perform many manual functions. Our instrumentation has been strictly evaluated by educators and state licensing boards. We are professionals.

Also, we are highly educated. Right now, dental assistants have few, if any, educational requirements. In some states, they don't even need a high school diploma to become a dental assistant. Hygienists, on the other hand, are college-degreed individuals. We have had rigorous training in either a bachelor's or an associate's program. We have paid our dues.

The number of hours hygienists spend in classrooms is exceedingly beneficial to the patient. Our knowledge of oral health, science, and dentistry is vital to help protect and inform the public. Every single day we point out our suspicions and recommendations to the dentist, who in turn bases her diagnosis on our assessment. Dentists and hygienists work together to provide the best care possible for our patients.

Dentists and hygienists are colleagues, not adversaries. Our goal is the same: to provide excellent dental care.

We know for a fact that our job is much more than cleaning teeth. If it were that simple, auxiliary personnel could step right in. But it's not so easy. There are thousands of hours of schooling and training under a dental hygienist's belt. We have learned what no one could in a dental office setting. We take what we've learned in the classroom, all of our classrooms, and apply it chairside. Auxiliary personnel cannot.

It's important to support our profession by supporting the ADHA. What hygienists want most, it seems, is to continue to have a great profession and earn a nice living. We can do that, but only if we practice maintenance.

Education Infatuation

Ann Battrell Stilwell, RDH, BS, an ADHA president, says that a graduate of an accredited dental hygiene program spends about 1,400 hours of classroom time studying sciences, academic subjects, and dental hygiene theory. That graduate will have an additional 600 hours of clinical instruction. Then, the graduate must pass a national written exam, regional written and clinical boards, and, finally, state jurisprudence, to obtain a license.

All this just to clean teeth?

The perception of some is that we are merely cleaning ladies. Flicking off calculus and polishing away stain, all the while chatting in a friendly manner with the patient. But we know our true value. We know it exceeds removal of calculus or coronal polishing. We have not merely learned a technical skill.

Preceptorship is a scary concept for any hygienist who fears losing her foothold in dentistry, and fears what may happen to patients. Preceptorship, a hygiene apprentice program, is a medieval throwback to the Dark Ages of dentistry. Simply teaching a person the technical skills needed to perform dental hygiene does not well serve the public. It could endanger public dental health. Patient safety is our main concern.

There are those who say that the monetary savings the public would receive would benefit society. It is difficult to imagine fees for prophys plummeting regardless of what type of individual is performing them. There are still overhead costs involved in running a hygiene department within a dental practice. It is unlikely the general public would receive any reduction in the cost of dental cleanings.

But the danger to their health could be enormous. It is frightening to think of an unlicensed auxiliary performing root planings or placing sealants. There are more to these functions than simply the manual skills involved. Unfortunately, the public is not aware of this. Luckily, most dentists are.

Most dentists appreciate the importance of proper dental hygiene performance. They understand the complexity of our profession. And they have a great appreciation for what a qualified dental hygienist can bring to their practice. We cannot risk alienating these dentists who support our profession.

We need to enlist them to further our careers. We cannot stand alone—we need the support of dentistry. We can show our value to their practices. One way to do that is to highlight the importance of dental hygiene education. Graduates of accredited hygiene programs are far superior as hygienists to any auxiliary personnel.

How can a waitress explain the complexities of periodontal disease and the need for root planing to her patient? Easy. She goes to an accredited dental hygiene school, graduates, passes the boards, and becomes a licensed dental hygienist. That's the only way to do it.

There has been a lot of talk about cutting the credit hours for dental hygiene education. Shortening dental hygiene programs could have disastrous results. We'd have graduating classes of half-hygienists.

The consensus still appears to be that offering an associate's or a bachelor's degree for dental hygienists gives women and men two wonderful choices. Since the dental hygiene clinical and classroom hours are the same, the programs are really identical, as far as the dental hygiene training is concerned. The exception is more extensive general academic classes for the bachelor's degree.

If this were a perfect world, it would be nice if dental hygiene programs could graduate all individuals with a bachelor's degree. Bachelor-degree programs offer a wealth of knowledge and breadth of education that all men and women should enjoy.

Unfortunately, time and cost deems this impossible. That's why dental hygiene as an associate's degree makes sense for certain individuals. Some say this is a move by dentistry to "keep us in our place." What we choose to believe depends upon our unique perspectives. For a lot of women and men, associate's degrees are their only viable chance at higher education. Bachelor's programs are preferable, but when the choice is no degree or associate's degree, it's more advantageous to have our society educated.

The move toward associate's degrees—in all fields, not just dental hygiene—is purely economic. Community colleges are enjoying a boom because education offered there is a value. Cost per credit hour is low compared with institutions offering a bachelor's degree, and education is still of a high caliber. They are wonderful institutions offering a solid education to many.

Also, one may attend a community college and still work full-time, which is difficult to do in a university setting. Some people who would never be able to attend a bachelor's program can obtain an associate's degree. Mothers with small children, or those of lower economic status can achieve a degree, just like those who are more fortunate or without family obligations. An entire set of people who could not attend college is now able. Associate's programs offer convenience with substance.

There are many hygienists today, perhaps your colleagues and friends, who would not have an RDH after their name if it weren't for the associate's program. We must remember that not everyone walks in the same shoes, and that judging others by our personal standards can be selfish as well as detrimental. There is a choice, and we should be thankful.

The important distinction is not between bachelor's and associate's, but between licensed hygienist and auxiliary.

Whether your degree is an associate's or a bachelor's, the important thing to remember that what is at issue is not a degree. The issue is the furthering of dental hygiene as a career for licensed dental hygienists. (For the record: I attended an associate's program in dental hygiene at New Hampshire Technical Institute three years after receiving my bachelor's in communications from Southern Methodist University.)

One of the devastating drawbacks to an associate's degree is the amount of time it takes to achieve said degree. What is billed as a two-year program takes a good three years to achieve. A three-year degree is like a "mini" bachelor's, and the graduate is not rewarded for the time he or she spends earning the certificate. Also, transferring credits toward a bachelor's program can be difficult or even impossible. More symbiosis should occur between bachelor's and associate's programs.

Education is the key issue on which we should focus. It is vital to the survival of dental hygiene as a profession—as well as promoting safe public dental health—that well-educated, licensed dental hygienists continue to perform hygiene-related functions. No one is served well by placing inexperienced, underqualified individuals in settings beyond their abilities. Our support of dental hygiene education will ensure its continuance.

Self-Regulation Regulated

First things first: self-regulation coupled with generalized supervision does not mean independent practice. Not all hygienists want independent practice, but most of us want generalized supervision. How many of us want self-regulation? And do we understand the implications of self-regulation on our profession?

Self-regulation, simply put, is a means by which hygienists would regulate themselves. We would regulate our professional duties, licensure, and education. Nurses, physical therapists, dietitians, cosmetologists and thousands of other licensed professionals have self-regulation. Dental hygiene is one of few who don't have it.

Most dentists lack desire to see hygienists achieve self-regulation because they don't see dental hygiene as a separate profession. They see dental hygiene as an extension of dentistry. To dentists, the profession of dentistry is like a connected bunch of grapes. Hygiene is a grape, but it is fully connected to the bunch, and cannot stand wholly apart. To dentists, hygienists can never be autonomous. We are part of dentistry.

The ADHA says the purpose of self-regulation is to protect the public. By ensuring only licensed healthcare individuals practice dental hygiene, we promote the safety and health of our patients. The worry is that dentists, who regulate hygiene, will push to have lesser-paid employees perform the tasks of dental hygienists. As they regulate, so they may take away. In other words, dentists have the final say in licensure of dental hygienists and which functions and procedures we may perform—or assistants may perform.

Dental hygienists are currently monitored by state dental regulatory boards. Boards are made up of dentists, hygienists, and consumers. Distressingly, there are more consumers on dental boards than dental hygienists on a nationwide basis. It makes one wonder how the needs of dental hygiene are served by boards composed mostly of dentists and consumers. This is worth pondering.

Dental boards create the rules for dentistry and dental hygiene in each state. They dictate which procedures assistants and hygienists can legally perform. They regulate dentistry and dental personnel through the rules of each state's dental practice act.

The ADHA is concerned that dentists are also dental hygiene employers and so can't make objective rules governing our profession. They might be controlled by economic rather than professional dictata. The organization feels that there might be a conflict of interest within the dental boards controlling dental hygiene. For instance, if a proposition suggests that dentists (employers) pay for half of the continuing education of dental hygienists, dentists (employers) would have an economic interest in seeing it put down.

Our hygiene organization is also concerned that dental hygiene issues may get lost in the shuffle when boards meet; dental boards are so concerned with dentistry, hygiene gets pushed aside. The ADHA believes that a dental hygiene board (made up of hygienists and consumers) would greatly benefit and promote the professional concerns of dental hygienists.

Would a dental hygiene board enact rules that would have dentists covering hygienists' continuing education costs and malpractice insurance fees? Would our board eliminate the associate's degree? Would our board push for expanded functions? Questions like these and others need to be asked and answered. The main purpose of a dental hygiene board should be to promote the profession of dental hygiene without alienating dental hygienists. A board of our own could help us create and define a workable path for the future of our profession. Self-regulation is something we all need to investigate and determine its feasibility in our individual states.

The ADHA

I am an active member of the ADHA. I carry a card in my wallet that tells me so. On the front is my name, social security number, membership information, and expiration date. On the back of this important-looking plastic card is the mission statement of the ADHA, a dental hygiene organization founded in 1923. Here it is, verbatim, courtesy of the ADHA:

Mission Statement

"To improve the public's total health, the mission of the American Dental Hygienists' Association is to advance the art and science of dental hygiene by increasing the awareness of and ensuring access to quality oral healthcare, promoting the highest standards of dental hygiene education, licensure and practice, and representing and promoting the interests of dental hygienists."

The ADHA legitimizes our stance as a profession related to, yet distinct from, dentistry. In other words, as dental hygienists we've got separate issues from those of dentists. The ADHA is the largest of all professional organizations for dental hygienists, and it services dental hygiene exclusively. There are other organizations vying for our membership, but the organization with the most members, the ADHA, has the economic and political means to see that our issues are addressed.

Without the ADHA we do not have a voice. Through this organization, we can nationally unite. The ADHA is our voice to promote the profession of dental hygiene.

For instance, if dentistry pushes for the expanded use of auxiliaries in preventive dentistry, we can speak out against it through the ADHA. It's our organization that represents our needs as a profession.

An association is nothing but a culmination of people. Whatever we want the ADHA to be, it will be. It's up to us, as members. If you like hygiene just the way it is (or even if you want to see it evolve differently), by joining and getting involved in the ADHA, your voice is heard. We're not going to agree on all issues, but united we stand stronger than we stand alone.

A man sat with his sons at the dinner table. They were all bickering. He asked the youngest son to fetch him some twigs. The son laid a bundle on the table in front of the man. "Sons, stop your fighting and listen. I want to see who can break this bundle in half." He passed the twigs around the table and each son tried to break the bundle, but couldn't.

The bundle was again in front of the man. With a knife he slit the rope tying the bundle, and the twigs separated. He passed a twig to each son. "Try to break it now, " he ordered. Each son easily broke his twig. "My sons," said the old man, "you are those twigs. Alone you are feeble and weak, but together, you are as the bundle—strong and unbreakable."

The same is true for dental hygienists. Alone we are vulnerable. We can be broken easily by those wishing to see us "stay in our place." But together we are hardy, unbreakable, and capable of many wondrous things.

On the back of my little plastic membership card is a list the of goals of the ADHA. Here they are, exactly as written:

Goals

- Maximize the utilization of the services of dental hygienists and to continue consumer advocacy in the healthcare delivery system.

- Promote the dental hygienist as a primary care provider of preventive and therapeutic services.

- Promote the self-regulation of dental hygiene education, licensure, and practice.

- Serve as the authoritative resource on all issues related to dental hygiene.

- Promote research relevant to dental hygiene.

- Increase membership and participation in the American Dental Hygienists Association.

- Provide for a viable financial base.

Participation in the ADHA will provide you with the benefits of furthering the profession of dental hygiene. Your voice can be heard, whether you agree with some or all of these statements. If you want to see changes in the ADHA, then involvement is a natural course. If you agree with the ADHA, and want it to continue, then your membership will keep it thriving.

The biggest show of support for the profession of dental hygiene is through the ADHA. Each membership in the ADHA is important and vital. Each membership makes the bundle that much stronger.

The Team?

Hygienists promoting the profession of dental hygiene do not need to alienate themselves from dentistry. Hygienists and dentists are in this dental boat together. We both desire the same goal: to provide excellent dentistry by helping general public dental health, and to make a nice living while doing so.

Dentists and hygienists can and do work together to give the patient the best dental care available. Dentists ensure restorative health, we ensure preventive maintenance. It's a symbiotic relationship that works well every day in dental settings nationwide.

Practice management gurus promote the term "team" to encompass all members of the dental office—business, assistants, hygienists, and dentists. They are striving for an atmosphere in the dental office that promotes better health-care delivery for the patient through team effort. It's as if we had all tried out for field hockey and were trying to take state championship. Indeed, sometimes the war between dentists and hygienists gets as rough as a field hockey match.

Yes, team is a word that works better at Wal-Mart than in dental offices. At Wal-Mart, there are no licensed snack bar saleswomen asserting self-regulation of hot dog sales. The corporate gurus teaching the team spirit may not have foreseen the complications of bringing that atmosphere to a health-care facility. In a health-care setting, a physician or dentist would never be a team player. They are providers and expected to produce, not pinch-hit or answer phones.

However, hygienists are expected to be team players, and at the same time be producers. This double standard could further antagonize the dentist/hygienist relationship. As licensed health-care workers, some dental hygienists are offended by the term team as it applies to their role in the dental office. Dental hygienists see themselves as a separate entity within the dental practice.

However, we must also see the view of the dentist. He wants harmony within his practice, and causing scathing discord may jeopardize our standing as a professional. Stating one's view and explaining it to others does not have to take on the appearance of war, and we do not have to play the "angry female" role. Debate is not hate. Debate is intellectual and noble. War is nasty and insipid, and unbecoming of a licensed health-care professional, whether dentist or hygienist.

> **Debate is not hate: intelligent, open discussion promotes dental hygiene.**

In opening up the lines of communication between hygienists and dentists we can pave the way for a better profession for everyone. Dental professionals who strive for war with dentists/hygienists are instigators. Instigators have no place in an intelligent discussion of the professions of dentistry and dental hygiene.

Our goals are not so polarized that we cannot forge a path of understanding and compromise that connects both parties. Dentists and hygienists should be partners in oral healthcare, not foes, and it's time for the banal squabbling to end and intelligent discussion to begin. It should be a challenge to us all to carry on a civilized debate regarding self-regulation of dental hygiene.

Chapter Eight

Back in the Saddle: Re-entering the Workforce or Switching Offices

"There is nothing in this world constant, but inconstancy."

—Jonathan Swift
from "A Critical Essay upon the Faculties of the Mind"

Charting Your Course

So you want the perfect hygiene position? Wouldn't it be nice if we could place ads and interview employers instead of vice-versa? I'd write mine as follows:

"Wanted: beautiful, multi-doctor dental office with large hygiene department, emphasis on perio health, sharp hygiene assistant, superior co-workers and yearly staff trips to Mexico, Hawaii, or the Caribbean. Must have health insurance plan, flexible hours, and great pay. Willing to work one night a week, one early morning a week, and one Saturday morning a month. Will not file or do paperwork, but will confirm patients, make appointments, and enter treatment plans. Please respond in writing to..."

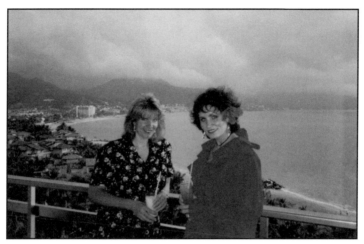

Fig. 8-1   Cat Schmidt and Cyd Ferris on a staff trip to Puerto Vallarta. Staff trips as bonuses are a benefit of employment at Gentle Dental.

That's my nirvana. Hey, wait, I've got that job! I guess it worked. I wrote my plan, and it came true. Now it's your turn. Write out your ideal job and then strive for it. You may be surprised at the results. (Fig 8.1.)

Take a blank piece of paper and divide it into two columns. Label one column necessities, and label the other desires. Then fill out your dreams. Do you absolutely, positively need weekends free? Write it under necessities. Would 10 a.m. be a nice starting time? Then place it under desires. Continue filling it out for a few days and let your mind wander on everything, including whether coffee is paid for by the office. (Fig. 8.2.)

Now it's time to write your want ad. No, don't place it in the local paper. Place it in your head. If you know ahead of time what you want, and what you'll accept, your job-hunting will be much more successful. It's impossible to reach a goal not set.

Compromise is okay in any position, as long as benefits make up the difference. I'll work that early morning (7 a.m.), which is a pain for me, because I like to write in the early mornings. I'd rather be at my computer than at the chair. But it's required, and I truly enjoy the rest of the job.

I will also work a late night (until 8 p.m.) because it doesn't bother me in the least. Actually, I chose to work two late nights, just so I could have Monday morning free. Ahh, compromise is good.

Necessities	Desires
weekends free	?$ pay
assisted probing/charting	full-time assistant
sick leave	salary vs. hourly
hour lunch	Wednesdays off
coffee and tea available	espresso machine
new equipment	two chairs

Fig. 8-2 Hygiene Job Requirements List

The Interview

The most important aspect to remember about an interview is that we are also interviewing our prospective employer. While she may think she's only testing us, we are giving her a thorough once-over, too. A successful interview has each participant investigating the other.

While we're researching our prospective employer, we're also checking out the office. We picture ourselves working there. Is it an atmosphere we feel comfortable in? We carefully inspect office personnel. We ensure there are no glaring personality differences that might cause clashes later on.

According to Elizabeth L. Post, granddaughter-in-law to the etiquette queen Emily Post, there are important rules to follow during an interview. Some of them are paraphrased here:[10]

1. Punctuality is a must.

Always be on time to an interview. You never want to keep an interviewer waiting, especially if the dentist has blocked time off his production schedule to see you. Be courteous of your future employer's (positive-thinking) schedule.

2. Shake hands when greeting and when leaving.

A firm, confident handshake will tell the interviewer more about you than you can imagine. This touching ritual is vital in business. It denotes trust and amicability. Both men and women should shake hands with confidence and strength.

3. Sit when asked, and keep correct posture.

Sit up straight and cross your legs at the ankles, not the knees. Never lean back or act too comfy in a chair. It will make you seem disinterested. By leaning forward and jutting your chin out, you present a picture of an interested party. It also makes one look thinner. Practice in front of a mirror so that it doesn't appear contrived.

4. Dress conservatively and nicely.

You'll want to look great, like on a first date, but not sexy. Polish your shoes, iron your blouse—whatever it takes to look your best. A good suit, pants with a blazer, or a skirt with a nice blouse will be perfect attire. Dress to impress.

5. Go alone, not with a friend or a group of interviewees.

You'll want to stand out in a crowd, not be a part of one. Don't go with other friends looking for the same position. You'll seem like a pack. Job hunting is a solo endeavor.

6. Take two extra resumes—one for you, one for interviewer.

You'll want one you can reference, and you'll want an extra one for the interviewer in case he can't locate yours. Also, he might want to pass it on to a colleague; you just never know where your next job is going to come from.

7. Speak clearly, confidently, and with good diction.

Speak up and don't act intimidated, even if you are. Remember Mary Kay Ash's words of wisdom, "Fake it until you make it." If you're asked a question, answer pleasantly but firmly. Wimps get wimpy jobs.

8. Know when it's time to leave; don't overstay your welcome.

Every interview takes a different amount of time, but if an hour has passed, start to head for the door. Usually the interviewer will drop subtle hints that time is up like, "I've really enjoyed talking with you," or, "It's nearly our lunch time." Pay attention to the clues.

9. Don't eat or drink, unless it's a lunch or breakfast interview.

Your interviewer will offer coffee or water, but it's just a nicety, you aren't really expected to accept. You'll want to keep your mouth free to talk.

10. Write a thank-you note and mail it within a day.

Thank-you notes to interviewers are your most important form of correspondence when job hunting, so take advantage of it. Also, it's proper etiquette.

In general, we just need to be on our best behavior during the interview process. We want to be the perfect applicant for the job. Our attitude should scream, "Hire me!"

Take your resume to a professional to typeset and revise. The ideal resume changes from year to year, and to have the best, go to the people who stay current in the job market. Do it right the first time, and your reward will be the position you desire.

Other job-hunting ideas include searching out employment headhunters. Headhunters are entering the health-care industry with rapid intensity. Check your area and make some calls. Perhaps a headhunter is what your city dictates. Remember, though, your interview at the headhunter's office should be taken as seriously as your interview with prospective employers. Headhunters spend their time on people they know will get the position. If you look like good material, you'll be promoted by the organization. Getting people hired is how headhunters make their commission, so a headhunter interview is a most important first step.

Another venue for job-hunting is to obtain a position with a temporary placement agency. Your interview here is vital, too. Temp work allows you flexibility, so if you've just moved, you'll have time to organize and settle into your new city. It also allows you to scope out different offices for possible employment, or check the local territory through different office gossip. Many permanent positions are filled with former temp employees. Employers prefer to hire people they know will fit the office.

Your perfect job may not come right away. You may need to go through a few different offices to find it. Your ideas of the perfect position may change as you understand the basics of working in many types of offices. A detriment may turn into an asset. The trick is to stick with it, and when you've found that perfect job, hold on tightly.

Showing our Worth

When we've gotten the job of our dreams, our next job is to keep it and enhance it. We'll want to sparkle in the eyes of our employer, so when the time comes for raises and bonuses, we're first in line. In proving our worth, our value rises. Remuneration is our reward.

We stand out at work by acting like the true professionals we are. We don't sit in the staff lounge sipping coffee and reading the paper when our patients fail their appointments—we stay busy. We get on the phone to reappoint the patient, we confirm our appointments, we sharpen instruments, or we clean our rooms. In effect, we're working when we're at work.

If we're hourly or salaried hygienists, then our employer must pay us whether we're with a patient or not. If we use our downtime to loaf, our employer will mentally note that she's paying us money to read *Newsweek*, her *Newsweek* at that. This is not the impression that wins raises and earns bonuses. This is an impression that may not provide us with job security.

If we're on commission, then our employer doesn't technically pay us for downtime. But he does expect us to be producing. It's in our best interest to stay productive and fill our chairs. Reading *People* will not help our production numbers, but confirming tomorrow's appointments will.

Another way to stand out as a professional at work is to keep personal phone calls at bay. Personal phone calls cause three detrimental events to our work life: they bother the receptionist; they tie up a business phone line; and they cut into our production time. Really, they're just bad practice.

Personal phone calls should be taken at home, not work.

In this day of voice mail and answering machines, there is no need to have our friends and family call us at work. We need to make a pact with kids or hubby to leave messages for each other on the home voice mail or answering machine. Friends should know our schedule so they may reach us at home.

By preventing needless phone messages—"May I take a message? She's with a patient"—we will offset any bad feelings from the person answering the phone, as well as our employer. We must never think that the receptionist will not speak to the employer if she feels she's become our personal secretary. The receptionist may not have the fortitude to confront us directly and ask that we cut down on our incoming personal phone calls. Instead, she may take her grievance directly to the employer, causing us to be the recipient of a reprimand.

Of course, emergencies are treated differently. If the situation is a true emergency, then we might need to be called away from the chair. But true emergencies don't include, "Billy took my toy," or, "Timothy asked me out, what should I wear?" We should remind those we love what constitutes an emergency and what doesn't.

To stand out as a professional at work, we must ensure that we look neat and clean and carry ourselves with confidence. It's an attitude that we adopt that encompasses our outer appearance and inner selves. Being a professional is to look and act the part. We feel better about ourselves, and our position in the office, if we conduct ourselves like true professionals (see Chapter 6).

Another way we can stand out at work is to carry our own weight. We should avoid the habit of relying on others to help us out. If it's our job, we should do it. The receptionist may have some free time one day to help us confirm patients, but we can't forget that she has her job, too. The next day she may be too busy to help, and yet too intimidated to tell us. This is common especially if others in the office are not as strong-willed as we are. It's easy to forget that assistants and receptionists may not have as much self-confidence as we possess.

If the receptionist gets bogged down by our work and is scared to tell us (hygienists can be a powerful bunch), her complaint will likely fall on the ears of the employer. He'll confront us, and soon we'll be busy explaining why the receptionist is doing our job. This is a situation to avoid from the get-go. We should do our own work.

Along those same lines, we must remember to mind our own business. Office gossip, while enticing, is extremely unprofessional, especially coming from a hygienist. We're licensed professionals who are expected to act differently than others in the office. Rumors can be ruinous and destructive.

One way to prevent their spread is to turn a deaf ear to office gossip. Gossip is usually inaccurate, always devious, and mostly harmful. People are never helped by rumors; they are only hurt. Promoting gossip is the antithesis of our professional duty, and it should be avoided at all costs. This includes gossip pertaining to other offices, other hygienists, and other dentists. Such rumors are rarely true and they are usually damaging.

Borrowing money or lending money is a definite no-no in the office, even to our "best friend." If we must get in a money situation with a friend, we are urged to make it a legal one—one with notarized papers signed by both parties. If we don't have proper, legal documentation of the loan, we might as well consider it a gift. Money has a way of splitting up friendships. It's a dangerous substance. The safest course is to steer clear of any money deals in the office.

Discussing our personal problems at work will probably make us the most unpopular co-worker, bar none. If someone has a sympathetic ear, we shouldn't take advantage of it. They may end up despising us in the end, because they've listened and listened and listened to our whining. Talking about our life is okay, but we should prevent ourselves from going overboard. Personal problems are just that: personal.

To ensure a good work environment, we should check our negative attitude at the door. No one likes to be around someone who's constantly complaining. So, the computers are down; big deal. So our patient didn't show; get over it. Keeping upbeat in the face of adversity is not only professional, but mature. Our employer notices negativity in her office staff; and if she doesn't, someone in the office will tell her about it. Maintaining a positive attitude is a habit to be developed. Getting rid of our negative attitude is like breaking a bad habit. In the long run, positive thinking keeps us happier, makes us like our work more, and, according to recent studies, will actually help to keep us healthy.

We need to keep track of the number of days we are absent. Maybe it's our third time this year, maybe it's our fourth. We have to know for sure, because our employer certainly does. Chronic absenteeism can be cause for dismissal. Also, if our employer has a different day count than we do, we have documentation at hand that can easily be verified by the appointment schedule.

Tardiness can also be a problem. Excessive tardiness can keep us from a raise or bonus. It could, like absenteeism, get us fired. We must ensure that we're always on time and ready to start the day or continue it (from lunch or dinner). Punctuality and professionalism go hand-in-hand. Our employer and our patients appreciate the effort.

Basically, having good manners and acting professional at work will help each of us maintain the job of our dreams. Maybe we'll even receive a raise or bonus because of our wonderful attitude. If we're unsure about whether it matters, we should think again. Employee raises and bonuses are subjective. We don't deserve them, we earn them. If our employers see us as deserving, we get them. If not, well...the picture is apparent. Our demeanor at work counts for everything, as there is little else about us that our employers can judge. Even if we don't achieve the bonus or raise, at the very least, we'll obtain a solid reference when searching for the perfect hygiene position.

Oceans of OSHA

Dental hygienists are in unique positions to aid the office in OSHA compliance. We have the educational background and intellectual ability, as well as the communication skills necessary for the job. Our employers would be wise to choose us to head their OSHA programs.

By taking on the task of implementing OSHA in our offices, we increase our worth to our present employer, and boost our esteem in a prospective employer's eyes. It's an asset as well as an outlet for us.

The time and effort are considerations, though. It is not an easy task, but a very rewarding one for the right candidate. The correct OSHA control manager needs to learn the ins and outs of preparing government forms and needs to understand how to read and decipher government documents. The candidate also has to be an interpreter to other staff members on the rules and regulations of OSHA. A good candidate is one that has a good rapport with other staff members, and one with whom the dentist could place trust.

A step-by-step guide to preparing an office for OSHA compliance is a great tool. In our office, we used one purchased from the ADA. It was extremely helpful in setting up our office regulations for both the BBP standard and hazard communications (hazardous chemicals). For more information on this and other OSHA guides, including an ADA tape series about OSHA, call the American Dental Association at (312) 440-2500.

Even with a step-by-step guide to implementing your OSHA program, there still is much to be done that doesn't fall into "filling in the blanks." For instance, an OSHA manager must write her own exposure control plan, map out work practice controls, train staff members yearly, train new staff members before they start work, and document everything from exposure incidents to HBV vaccines. There is enough work to do when starting out that it practically takes a full-time employee to complete it. However, once it's in place, the upkeep is easier, but vitally necessary.

It's worth considering accepting this responsibility. Dental hygienists are naturally suited for this work. There is much support out there, too, from all sorts of sources including your state OSHA office and the national OSHA office. Becoming your office's exposure control manager can be a very rewarding experience.

Annie, Annie, Are You OK?

In our office, all employees who work directly with patients are certified in cardiopulmonary resuscitation (CPR). That's about 22 people a year to train. While it's an important and valuable function, it's time consuming and expensive. It really adds up when one hires two instructors, rents a few mannikins, and buys certification cards for the entire office.

That's when Schmidty (my dad) got a brainstorm.

"Hey, Cat, why don't you become a CPR instructor? Then you could teach us all."

I thought, oh, why not? So, I contacted a local ambulance station that teaches the instructors' course to emergency medical technicians. The woman who answered the call said, sure come on down to the station and fill out the forms. She signed me up and I was ready for the class.

The course I participated in took one day. It was similar to a lengthened CPR certification class containing a more expansive written test. The training was intense but enjoyable. Afterwards, I was certified to teach CPR to health-care providers, which meant I could then teach everyone in the office. Everyone, including the dentists.

We rent the mannikins from the local American Heart Association, and buy certification cards and materials from the state office in Des Moines. I'm not sure how much it has saved on cost—probably some—

but the time factor for employees has been extremely beneficial. I block off time on my schedule and sit around in our denture reception area, waiting for employees to approach me when they have time to perform the physical test. They can take the written exam at any time during the two days we execute CPR certification.

It helps everyone out, because they're allowed to play with the mannikins and really get a feel for it, instead of hurrying through a course at a hospital or an office. And I'm available for two mornings, so no one has to come in and get certified on their day off. (In our office, we work four days a week, having one weekday free.)

You might consider acquiring CPR certification to teach healthcare providers. The day-long class for those who already possess CPR certification is not much more difficult than the regular classes we take each year. It can be a boost to your resume and a benefit to your employer.

In the Public Eye

Anytime we are out in the public as dental hygienists, we are promoting dentistry. In most dental offices, we field calls from schools, daycares, libraries, and all sorts of places asking that a hygienist visit. These are perfect opportunities to promote dental hygiene, oral healthcare, and your dental office.

If it's something you enjoy doing, I urge you to not only do it, but to promote it. Let your employer know what you're doing. Put it on your resume. In other words, get credit for your actions. Why not? You're working hard, so reap some rewards from it.

Like a lot of offices do, we print our name and phone number on each toothbrush. Ask your employer if you can take them with you for a treat for the kids. Everyone loves to get a present, and what's better for a hygienist to hand out than toothbrushes?

Does your dentist have visual aids you can bring to your engagement? Maybe if your employer knew what you were doing, she'd purchase some equipment for you. Getting her business name in the public, through you, should be worth a little investment. "This is Vera from Gentle Dental. She's here to talk to us about brushing our teeth."

If you're out there doing good deeds, teaching children (and adults) about good oral hygiene, don't be ashamed to receive accolades for it. You deserve it.

Every other month I write a column, called "Ask Your Dental Hygienist," in a local seniors magazine. I share the column with Schmidty, who writes "Ask Your Dentist" every month I'm not published. My column is fun, and it promotes dental hygiene and dental issues, such as fluoride, recalls, and gum disease. It's my way of giving to the community, in a manner I'm comfortable with.

Speaking in front of groups is enjoyable, but not nearly so enjoyable for me as writing a column. You don't have to speak, or give brushing instructions to preschoolers. Ask yourself, what are my strong suits? And take it from there. Meshing your career and your hobby can be a blast.

Expanding Functions

One of the best ways to spice up your resume is by becoming certified in expanded functions. In the states where expanded functions are legal, your services will be appreciated. These are abilities you bring to the practice that aid your employer and make his life easier, and make you all the more valuable.

For a dentist who doesn't have to break away from his patient to IJ your patient, life is easier. He knows you're capable, as you've obtained the training and certification, and he appreciates the time you save him.

If your state does not allow expanded functions, consider pushing for such legislation. Check with your local and state hygienists' associations, and join their efforts. We promote our profession by expanding the duties of dental hygienists. When we allow our profession to grow by the introduction of expanded functions, we are promoting dental hygiene for the public good.

Perhaps your strength lies in your abilities to champion dental hygiene causes. Go for it. Expanded functions are not the only issues at the state and local levels. Some areas are still trying to get general supervision. Others are battling preceptorship. Still others are fighting to keep hygiene job duties assignable only to licensed dental hygienists. There are insurance issues, legal issues, self-regulation, and a multitude of other issues facing our profession. There are issues pertaining to individual states, as well as national issues to be faced by all dental hygienists.

Whatever the topic, if you're legislatively inclined, you're sure to find a cause to champion. Embrace and advocate it. You may even find a new career, or, at the very least, a resurgence of dental hygiene pride.

Postscript

Coffee Breaks:
Taking Time for You

"How many cares one loses when one decides not to be something, but to be someone."

—Coco Chanel,
remark.

Daytimer Dreaming

Bobbie wrote the time in bold, red numbers in her Daytimer. Then she used the marker to copy the same time onto her husband's Daytimer, albeit using smaller strokes. Lastly, she wrote the time onto the family's refrigerator calendar.

There. It was done.

Bobbie sat down at the desk in the kitchen and pulled out a stack of bills. A guilty feeling crept over her. She glanced at numbers she had written on a list on the refrigerator door. On Friday afternoon, from three until five o'clock, Bobbie was occupied. What would her family say?

"Mom, do we have any ice cream?" asked her 10-year-old son Josh.

"I think so. Check the freezer." She punched some numbers into the calculator.

"Yuck, it's peppermint. Don't we have any good kinds?"

Bobbie put the bills aside and walked over to her son, whose head stuck into the frosty air.

"There's some popsicles, and a fudge bar left," she said reaching for the boxes.

"No! I want chocolate ice cream. Can't you go to the store?"

Bobbie took a deep breath and felt her neck muscles tighten. She slowly let out the air and tried to relax her aching shoulders.

"No, I can't go to the store." She glanced at the bills on the desk, then mentally planned a trip to the dry cleaners on her way to pick up Heidi from gymnastics.

Her son stormed out of the kitchen. She sighed.

Later, her husband thumbed through his daytimer to find a phone number.

"What's this on Friday?" he demanded.

She had forgotten all about it.

"You're going to be busy from three until five?"

"Umm, yes." Hey, that sounded good, Bobbie thought. She felt stronger, taller, so added, "Yes, I am."

"And you'll be doing...?" He rotated his hand, expecting her to fill in the blank.

"I've got plans."

Her husband looked at her quizzically. "You're not having an affair, are you?"

She laughed. "And put it in my husband's Daytimer? I'm not stupid, Kevin."

He smiled. "I don't get it. What's Friday about?"

"Time for me. Time to myself."

"Oh, man, not more of those books again. Geez, Bobbie, that pop psychology stuff is a bunch of bull——,"

Heidi walked into the room.

"——oney," he finished.

Bobbie didn't want to turn this into another fight. She was too tired to fight.

"Kevin, it's not going to interfere with your schedule. I just wanted you to know that I won't be available."

"Whatever," he said curtly, and scribbled down the number he needed.

Bobbie bit her tongue. She hated it when Kevin didn't understand she needed things that were just hers, and hers alone. Time to be herself. Not a wife, not a mother, just Bobbie. He dismissed these things as foolish, but to Bobbie they were important.

Two years ago she had entered a painting class. It had always been a dream of hers to be an artist. She was praised in high school for her drawings. But then came dental hygiene school, and marriage, and the kids. Her artist-self slipped into obscurity. Kevin had teased her unmercifully about the painting class, but she had stuck with it. Her artistic ability emerged beautifully. Eventually, even Kevin complimented her work.

But as the kids grew older, their lives became much more hectic. Even with a three-quarter-time hygiene position, time was still like gold. Soon, being a chauffeur, mother, cheerleader, chaperone, head cook, and all the other titles she bore was just too much. She hadn't had time in months to paint.

That's when Bobbie decided to schedule time for herself. If I don't do it now, she thought, when am I going to? She learned in church that God gives everyone certain, wonderful talents. If you don't use them, you may lose them. She didn't want to lose her painting ability. She wanted to use it.

Thus the red marker and the times—"3:00 to 5:00—Bobbie"— written boldly on all calendars. She always said, when I get a free hour I'll get out my watercolors. Well, a free hour never came. And, she knew, it never would. Unless she did something about it.

All week long Bobbie fought for her two hours on Friday. Josh said since it wasn't a real appointment, she shouldn't mind taking him out to the Snyder Farm. "I'm busy," she replied. Heidi insisted her life would be ruined if they didn't go shopping on Friday for a new outfit for the party that night. "I'm busy," she replied. Even Kevin joined in, but she kept repeating throughout the week, "I'm busy."

It wasn't easy, and it took real effort. Everyone assumed that because they weren't "real" plans, that she would drop them at a moment's notice. But she knew that if she did, that free hour for her painting would be a pipe dream, and she would never get to paint.

Bobbie held fast, even through pressure at work.

"We're going out after work on Friday, why don't you come?"

"I'm busy."

"You never come. Can't you change your plans just this once?"

The intimidation bothered her. But she didn't give in. She knew they were playing childish games by coercing her into joining them. Bobbie's plans were set in stone.

On Friday, Bobbie gathered up her easel and accessories, packing them in the trunk. She filled a cooler with water, soft drinks, and some crackers. She grabbed the boom box, a Mozart CD, and spare batteries, and headed out into the countryside in her Jeep.

The day was lovely; it was late spring and the earth was coming to life. Bobbie found a restful place by a stream where a budding forest met the flower-speckled plains. She captured the afternoon on paper and in her soul.

Taking Time For You

Time is a commodity. Like soap, sugar, and soybeans, it can be bought and sold—probably not on the commodities market, but similarly, in our minds. When we make plans we sell our time to others. When we schedule time for ourselves, we buy time.

Our society is oddly fast-paced. One would think with all the technological advances in the last century, there'd be more free time, not less. However, it's rare to find a day, or even an hour, with nothing to do. Seems like there's always something—washing, cleaning, errands, job, school, kids, significant other. How many times can you hear, or say, "There's just not enough time in a day?"

It's true. But it doesn't have to be depressing. We can get a handle on it. We can have our cake and eat it, too, as long as we're willing to compromise. Let's say we want a couple hours to read a book and take a bath. No interruptions. Sounds delicious. All we have to do is schedule it, just like Bobbie did.

The sky won't fall and the world won't end if we're away for a couple of hours. Kids will cry and moan and complain. They're kids. They're egocentric. They aren't really suffering. I knew a woman who hired a babysitter just so she could take naps in the afternoon. She left strict orders not to be disturbed. It worked for her.

The trick is finding out what you want, and how to get it to fit into your life. If you need an afternoon to go shopping by yourself, then you should schedule it. Write it onto your calendar as if it were a real appointment. After all, it *is* a real appointment. It's an appointment with a very important person: YOU!

As health-care professionals, we're natural givers. We give to our patients, co-workers, and employers. At home, we give to our families and friends. Where do *we* fit in? Hopefully, we haven't lost our own place on our list of importance. We're important and worthy individuals, deserving of attention and time.

> It is not selfish to desire time for ourselves;
> in fact, it's just the opposite.

Scheduling alone time is the epitome of generosity. It is a very giving and loving thing to do for ourselves, and for those who join in our lives. It's a present we give, and receive. Everyone around us benefits.

In recharging our batteries, we make ourselves more vital, more energetic, and better people. Time alone—engrossed in a favorite project, book, nap or bath—helps restore our vigor. We emerge refreshed and rejuvenated.

We are calmer and happier people. Friends and family like us more. We don't snap at co-workers and we don't get frustrated with difficult patients. We are restored like the ceiling of the Sistine Chapel—vibrant, remarkable and stunning.

But, what's this, no time? Someone once said, if it's important enough, I'll make time for it. We just need to realize the importance of taking care of ourselves. How can we take care of so many others if we're not taking care of ourselves? A good question to ponder.

Maybe we need to pull a few minutes from here or there. Maybe we need to give up an activity. Maybe the laundry doesn't need to be folded as if ready for inspection by an army sergeant. Maybe other people can do some of the tasks we take on so willingly. Maybe we can make the time.

Yes, there will be people who do not understand. There will be people close to us that will not support us. What we need to question is not our desire for time for ourselves, but others' reactions. Why are they threatened by our need for time to read a book, paint a picture, watch a movie, or sit by a fire?

Perhaps they are concerned that they will lose something we give them, such as cooking meals, running errands and taking phone messages. We can reassure them that things will get done. We can ask them to perform the tasks. We can tell them, nicely, that this is just the way it's going to be, and they'll have to get used to it.

Perhaps they are worried they will lose us. We can reassure them that this will make us like them more, not less. We can show them we love/like them, but we need to be on our own, too. If they persist, even after assurances, we must resign ourselves to the fact that it's their problem, not ours. They will have to work on it by themselves. We've done and said all we can.

The only sure way to obtain the time you need is to schedule it. Make a commitment to yourself the way you would to someone else. Write it down, and don't go back on your word. Treat it as an important event, because it is. You deserve it. Take a stand for yourself.

An International Coffee Moment

It sounds ridiculous. We see the commercial—the two women sipping a coffee concoction, quietly smiling while enjoying themselves. It's nearly a cliché. But, wouldn't it be nice just to sit for a moment during the day and drink flavored coffee? Or, at least put your feet up and relax, not thinking about your next patient or your last? A real break.

We have them in our office every now and then, and it's wonderful. Sometimes it involves making a pot of flavored coffee and standing by the coffeemaker idly chit-chatting. Other times, someone will have made brownies (no small feat in an office of 40), and there will be groups, at different times, in the staff lounge snacking on brownies, lounging on the couch or at the table.

It's important during the workday to schedule breaks. Hygiene is an intense vocation, both mentally and physically demanding. Breaks are necessary to keep ourselves fresh. Think of what means most to you—like taking a brisk walk, eating a treat, calling a friend, or reading a magazine—and plan it into your day.

Two hygienists in our office have begun getting fat-free strawberry shortcake ice cream waffle cones in the afternoons. Mmmmm. I prefer the flavored coffee route and gabbing by the coffee counter. Some in the office walk around the building or, when it's nice, across the street to a park brimming with flowers.

The important thing is that it gives you a break from your routine, just like recess did for us in school. Whatever you do, do something different from your job for a few minutes each day. When you come back, you'll be better focused and more alert.

> **Breaks are like recess. They're a scenic detour in the road of our day.**

By no means do breaks have to happen at work. If it's just impossible to get a break at work, take one directly after work. Stop by a coffee house, park, gym, or frozen yogurt place on your way home. Plan a moment or two of restful meditation in the operatory or staff lounge once you're done for the day. Anything will work, just set your imagination free. (Fig. 9.1.)

---

1. Plan a lunch date with friend in the middle of the day. Meet for a quick bite somewhere near the office, but not in the office.
2. Take a walk arount the block, or to a local store to buy a soda. If there's a park nearby, stroll through it and fill your lungs with fresh air.
3. Bake muffins for the entire office and bring in orange juice, milk, colorful napkins, and paper plates. Make any day a special occasion.
4. Go to a florist shop and idly spend time savoring the scents and looking over the bric-a-brac. Buy some flowers for no reason, for the office or for your home.
5. Set a timer for three minutes, Sit comfortably with your eyes closed. Let your mind wander, maybe picturing an exotic locale or favorite place. When the buzzer goes off, poof!, you're back at work.

Figure 9.1 Ideas for Hygiene Success

Breaks at home are equally important. Sometimes it's easy for us to forget that home is where we relax. There's so much to do there—iron, wash, clean, rake, vacuum, fold, neaten, cook, fix—the list goes on and on. We need to remember to take time to enjoy our home life. Home is where the heart is, our heart.

A friend of mine kept her romance novels in the bathroom, and when she just needed time away from everybody and everything, she'd slip into the john and read. She said she'd lie on the shaggy rug in there and pull out her novel. A few pages for a few minutes and she felt rejuvenated. And who's going to say anything about being in the bathroom?

> **When we're not at work,**
> **we need to remember to take time to relax.**

References

1   Schmidt, Duane A. *Iowa Pride* Ames, IA: Iowa State University Press, 1996.

2   Schmidt, Duane A. *Schmidt's Anatomy of a Successful Dental Practice*, Tulsa, OK: PennWell Publishing, 1996.

3   *"Dental Economics"* June 1997, Vol. 87, No. 6: 55.

4   "ADHA Position Paper on Managed Care," 1996.

5   *"Access"* May-June 1997, Vol. 11, No. 5: 35-43.

6   McKenzie, Maria. *"Access"* May-June 1997, Vol. 11, No. 5: 37.

7   Offenbacher, Katz, Fertik, Collins, et. al. "Periodontal infection as a possible risk factor for preterm, low birth weight." *Journal of Periodontology*, 1996.

8   Love, Susan, MD. *San Francisco Examiner*, as quoted by Joy Rothke, 3/27/97, Section C: 1, 11.

9   All people in this book are real; however, they have been renamed and moved to different states for the author's amusement, and—oh, yeah—for their privacy.

10 Post, Elizabeth L. *Emily Post's Etiquette*, New York: Harper-Collins Publishers, Inc, 1992.

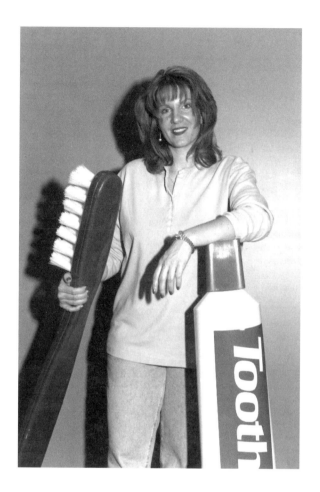

About the Author

Cat Schmidt lives and works in eastern Iowa. She is one of six full-time hygienists at Gentle Dental, a practice owned by her father, Dr. Duane A. Schmidt. She is a CPR instructor and the office exposure control manager for OSHA programs. She received her bachelor's in communications from Southern Methodist University and her associate's in dental hygiene from New Hampshire Technical Institute. When not "chairside," she loses herself in novels and travels the globe seeking adventure and mystery.

Index

A

Absenteeism..146
Abusive behavior 107–109
Accusations 30–32
ADA 34–35, 38–40
    codes 34–35
ADHA........................39–40, 68, 127–129, 132–136
    goals..135
    team practice 136-137
Aging population 85–90
American Arbitration Association 28, 30
American Dental Association. SEE ADA.
American Dental Hygienists' Association. SEE ADHA.
Americans with Disabilities Act..87
Arbitration 27–30
Asset coverage 25–27
Assistance vs. assistants..80–81
Associate's degree..129–132
Attitude change 111–115

B

Baby boom population..84–85
BBP standard 46–49, 54–57, 60
    compliance..46–49
    hygienist's rights 54–55
    training 60
Binding arbitration..27–30
Biohazards 52
Blood and other potentially infectious materials. SEE BOPIM.
Bloodborne pathogen standard. SEE BBP standard.
BOPIM 46, 56, 59

C

Cameras 17
Capitation patients..40
Cardiopulmonary resuscitation. SEE CPR TRAINING
Centers for Disease Control and Prevention 62
Chartit 5
Code blue..102–103
Code red..103
Code yellow 102–110
Codes (insurance) 34–35
Coffee breaks 156–158

Index

Compliance methods 58
Computers 1-24
   breakdown 22-24
   electronic dental office...8-19
   repair 22-24
   speed..19-20
   timing..19-20
   training..2-3,5-6
   World Wide Web 20-22
Computer–digitized radiography 3, 12, 93
Conservative dress..142
Course of treatment...33
Co–worker relationships 115–119, 145–146
CPR training 148–149

D
Definitions 56–57
Dental care market...79
Dental hygiene training 129–132
Dental insurance 32–34
Dentist/hygienist relationship 121–123
Dentists' needs..123–127
Direct reimbursement 41–42
Disposal methods..59
Disruptive patients...102–110
Documentation 30–32
Drug–related conditions 87

E
E–mail 20–21
Education...129–132
Electronic dental office SEE COMPUTERS
Employer problems 115–119
Engineering controls 56, 58
Erratic behavior 107–109
Exclusive provider organization 37
Expanded functions...150
Explosion codes..6–7, 35
Exposure control plan 57–58, 60
Exposure incident 56
Exposure control 56–60

F
Fee for service 35–36, 41

Female–friendly office 93–94
Financial stage (computerization) 8
Four–handed hygiene 79–80
Full mouth series 3

G
Geriatric patients 83–94
   aging population 85–90
   changing patient needs 83–84
   Medicare 84–85
   women's oral needs 90–93
Gingivitis 92
Gossip 145–146

H
Handicapped–accessible dental care 87
HBV 57, 59–60
   vaccination 59–60
   symptoms 60
Health issues 51–52
Health maintenance organization 37
Hepatitis B virus. SEE HBV.
HIV 46, 57
Holistic medicine 87
Home care education 90–92
Hormonal factors 90–92
Hormone replacement therapy 92
Housekeeping 59
Human immunodeficiency virus. SEE HIV.
Hygiene and dentistry synthesis 121–137
   dentists' needs 123–127
   education 129–132
   hygienists' needs 127–129
   profitability 123–127
   RDH vs. DDS 121–123
   self regulation 132–133
Hygiene assistance 67–81
   assistance vs. assistants 80–81
   four–handed hygiene 79–80
   hygiene assistants 68–72
   office as assistant 72–76
   tasks 69–70, 77, 79–81
   trends 67–68
   two-chair hygiene 76–78

Hygiene assistants 68–72
Hygiene department profitability...123–127
Hygienist scheduling 72–73
Hygienist's tasks/duties 72–77
Hygienists' needs 127–129

I

Independent practice 132–133
Individual practice association 37–38
Infection protection 45–65
    BBP standard 56–57
    compliance methods 58
    exposure control 56
    exposure control plan 57–58
    HBV vaccination 59–60
    housekeeping..59
    inspection results..55–56
    inspection preparation..54–55
    latex allergy 60–63
    OSHA..45–47
    OSHA improvements..64–65
    OSHA inspection 49–54
    OSHA inspection request 64
    personal protective equipment 58–59
    teamwork..47–49
    training 60
Insurance information 15
Insurance/legal issues 25–44
    arbitration 27–30
    codes 34–35
    dental coverage 32–34
    direct reimbursement 41–42
    documentation..30–32
    malpractice insurance 25–27
    managed care 37–41
    patient payment options 35–36
    social insurance 42–44
Internet 20–22
Interview rights (OSHA) 54–55
Interview (job hunting)..141–143
    speech habits 142

J

Job evaluation 139–141

Job hunting 139–143
Job interview 141–143

L
Language barrier 100–101
Latex allergy...60–63
Legal counsel 52–53
Legal issues 8
Liability 25–27
Litigation 25–27
Logistics 64

M
Malpractice insurance 25–27
Managed care..37–41
Mannerisms/language 95–97
Medicare...84–85
Menopausal women...92
Money borrowing/lending 146
Mouse (computer) 23

N
Nursing home patients 83, 87

O
Occupational Safety and Health Administration. SEE OSHA.
Office as assistant...72–76
Office politics...115–119
Off–limits conversation 98
Off–site dental hygiene 83
Online services..20
Oral care..87
Oral conditions charting 93
Oral conditions (geriatric).....................................85–90
Oral health future 83–84
Orange alert 103
OSHA compliance 147–148
OSHA improvements 64–65
OSHA inspection 49–54, 64
    request for 64
OSHA program director..49
OSHA training 60
OSHA 45–47, 49–54, 60, 64–65, 147–148

Osteoporosis...92–93
Over–compliance 47

P

Partial computerization 8–9
Partial dentures 86
Patient care form 11–16, 99–100
Patient care plan 109–110
Patient communication 74, 78, 90–92, 97–100, 102–110
Patient complaints 30–32
Patient interaction..............................30–32. SEE ALSO Code yellow.
Patient needs changing 83–84
Patient payment options 35–36
Patient scheduling...9–11, 17, 97–98
Patient treatment plan 17–18, 33
Periodontal debridement 16
Periodontal disease 89
Periodontal screening and recording..16
Personal protective equipment 56, 58–59
Personal phone calls 144–145
Personal problems 146
Personal relationships 115–119
Personal time 154–156
Physician–hospital organization 37–38
Point–of–service plan...37–38
Politics/sex/religion 98
Position entry–change 139–150
    CPR 148–149
    expanded functions 150
    interview 141–143
    OSHA 147–148
    Posture..142
    professional behavior..144–147
    public relations 149–150
    Preceptorship...129
    strategy...139–141
    Preferred provider organization...............................37–38
Pregnancy..91–92
Preventive dentistry 37
Preventive maintenance..136
Prioritization 69–70
Professional behavior...144–147
Professionalism 95–119, 144–147
    mannerisms/language 95–97

words 97–100
thank you..110–111
attitude change 111–115
personal relationships 115–119
total package 119
behavior..144–147
Profitability 39, 72, 123–127
profit margin 39
Public relations 149–150
Punctuality..141

Q
Quoting fees...15–16

R
RDH vs. DDS 121–123
References 159
Regulated waste 56
Restorative dental care...136
Resumes 142, 150

S
Safety issues...52
Safety/health hazard complaints 49–53
Scheduling time 151–154
break time 156–158
Self–assessment 111–115
Self–regulation 132–133
Signatures (computer) 11
Smoking..58
Social insurance 42–44
Speech habits 95–97
Strategy 139–141

T
Tardiness 146
Team practice 136–137
Teamwork..47–49
Third–party lenders 35–36
Third–party prepayment 35–36
Threatening behavior..107–109
Time management 151–158
scheduling time 151–154
time for yourself 154–156

scheduling breaks 156–158
Timing an interview...142
Timing (computer) 19–20
Title XIX program 42–44, 109–110
Tooth loss..88
Total package 119
Training issues 60
Treatment alteration...109–110
Treatment plan...104–107
Trends (hygiene assistance)...67–68
Two–chair hygiene 76–78

U
Universal precautions 57–58, 62
Unsafe work practices 45
Usual, customary, and reasonable fee 36

W
Welfare patients 42–44, 109–110
Women's oral needs 90–92
Words (professionalism) 97–100
Work area layout 76–80
Work environment safet, ...49–53
World wide web..20–22